PALEO DIET
FOR STUDENTS

2 Books in 1: PALEO Diet GUIDE for Beginners: An easy guide to the with over 200 Delicious Quick and Easy Recipes.

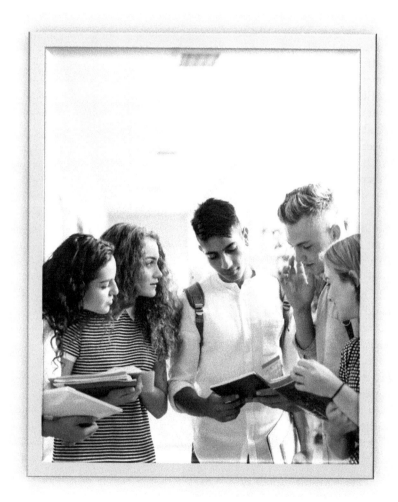

By

Robert Baker

TABLE OF CONTENT

PART I: INTRODUCTION

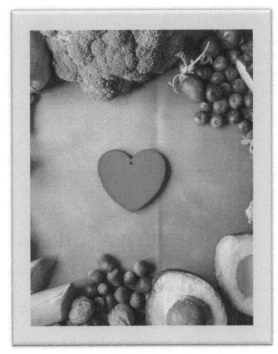

The paleo diet is said to rid you of migraines, get rid of bloating, eliminate seasonal allergies, clear up acne, and shed a few pounds. In addition, natural foods in appropriate portions help you feel reasonably satisfied, as they help keep blood sugar levels even and hunger hormones well balanced.

Top paleo guidelines for starters:

Skip all grains (both whole and refined), dairy, packaged snacks, legumes, and sugar in favor of vegetables, fruits, meats, eggs, seafood, nuts, fats, seeds, and oils - sounds easy, however, going cavewoman successfully takes common sense. You can follow these principles of the paleo diet, for starters.

IDENTIFY MOTIVATION

Most individuals turn to the paleo diet to help with medical issues, such as GI problems, allergies, and autoimmune conditions. Some need to feel good on a day-to-day basis or believe it is a healthy way to eat. Your main reason will help you determine the guidelines to follow and what you need to be meticulous about. Also, be strict about your principles for the first month. That is enough time to start noticing good changes in your health.

CLEAN UP THE KITCHEN

Collect all the "no" foods from the paleo diet list, such as packaged foods, cereals, milk, cereals, cheese, vegetable oils, yogurt, and beans, and throw them in the dust bin. Doing all of the above has one advantage: it's easy to avoid temptation when it's not there. But in case you like to take small steps at first, then it works too. For example, you can probably cut out dairy during the first week, remove refined grains in the second week, skip grains during the third week, and so on until you follow the paleo diet. Either way, be sure to buy whole foods; then, you have a lot of work to design your paleo diet meal plan.

Follow the 85/15 approach

After the first 30 days, several experts suggest the 85/15 rule, which means that 85% of the time you are strictly following the paleo diet, leaving 15% for non-paleo, whether it's a granola bar (which you could opt for the paleo granola recipe), a burger (bun and all) at the barbecue, or some cocktails. Next, focus on how you feel after introducing new things to the paleo diet. For example, when you eat a scoop of delicious ice cream and wake up bloated the next day, you may decide that the future discomfort is not worth it.

COOK

Since the paleo diet is based on fresh, whole foods, it's easy to prepare meals at home rather than at a restaurant where it's difficult to control the ingredients. So, take this golden opportunity to experiment with new foods - it might be a bit challenging for you to buy strange-looking vegetables at the market and ask the shopkeeper for advice on how to cook them perfectly.

You could also search online or invest in a paleo diet cookbook for inspiration, so the meals stay tasty and aren't just plain chicken breasts along with simple carrots and cabbage.

Expect 1 setback (or 2)

It is normal to follow the paleo diet and fall back into the usual eating habits. It's a good learning process.

You can also look for like-minded people who are already following this diet through local forums, groups, blogs, and Facebook and connect with them for assistance to keep you on track and save you.

THE LABEL DECODER

As you know, don't eat donuts, crackers, and cookies, but some foods are not paleo: nut butter jars, peanut butter (this is a legume); nuts along with added sugars; and lunch meats, malt vinegar, soy sauce, and other sauces and marinades (some consist of sugar, soy, preservatives, and gluten). So be sure to see the entire ingredient list as you purchase anything in the package.

Think about your plate

You're taught to always reserve half your plate for vegetables, a quarter for lean protein, and a quarter for whole grains. But, as you transition to the paleo diet, stop saving a spot for grains:

The balanced plate contains a palm-sized protein, a tablespoon of fat, and veggies, veggies, veggies (fill the remaining container with these).

CHANGE YOUR OIL

Rather than reaching for corn, canola, or soybean oil for frying, you'll want to use lard or coconut oil. Seriously. These good-quality saturated fats are good for preparing food because they are stable and don't oxidize during heating (oxidation also releases harmful free radicals).

When it comes to lard, animal fats - in the case of grass-fed cows - have been packed with large amounts of omega-3s and a form of fat known as conjugated linoleic acid that some studies find could help burn fat.

Some dietitians also suggest butter from grass-fed cows; however, many limit dairy products of all kinds. (The choice is all yours.) For cold applications, you can use nut oil, olive oil, and avocado oil.

EATING MEAT

Many people have restricted meat from the paleo diet because they believe it's terrible for your health. You can also eat meat, but make sure it is high quality. So, you can say goodbye to processed meats that include bologna, hot dogs, and salami.

Wild meats such as bison, wild boar, and elk are an excellent choice for you, followed by pasture-raised poultry and meats, and lean grain-fed meat should be the last choice. And, for seafood, choose wild-caught often, and low mercury and sustainable choices are best.

You can easily make your sweet tooth go crazy.

Removing sugar is a primary daunting task for many people at first. But, in case you love to have a treat right after dinner, then you can swap your cookies or just for you with a piece of fruit. (For your sugar cravings, experts say the paleo diet allows for dried mangoes).

Over time, your taste buds will adjust accordingly, and that Oreo you loved so much before may become so much sweeter for you now. Seriously, it can happen!

YOU CAN EAT OUT

A few business dinners and brunches with best friends are possible with a paleo diet. All it takes is a little bit of ingredient research. But, first, you need to take a look at your menu ahead of time and choose 1 or 2 options that you could paleo-size.

This can be wild salmon and broccoli. (Also, request twice as many vegetables rather than rice pilaf.) Also, in a restaurant, don't be ashamed to ask pertinent questions about the things being prepared and request changes if necessary.

WHOLE FOODS THAT ARE RICH IN NUTRIENTS

If the food is not in the state it was in when it was pulled from the earth, then there is an excellent chance that it has been refined and is not optimal. By selecting food directly from nature, our bodies receive those nutrients needed to heal our bodies.

Avoid nutrient-poor, processed and refined foods that are made in factories.

I meant pasteurized dairy products, grains, seed oils (canola, cottonseed, corn, and soybeans), artificial sweeteners, and refined sugar (fructose corn syrup). Most of these foods take nutrients away from the body for digestion, which negates eating, which is to nourish a human body and the nutrients to grow and repair itself.

Yes, it would take some time to learn the paleo lifestyle. There might be some confusion at first as you work to change your shopping habits, eating out, and meal preparation; therefore, this is vital to switch to a gradual pace that fits perfectly. Also, be aware that more "non-paleo" foods need to be reworked to fit the paleo lifestyle.

EATING FOR A HEALTHY DIGESTIVE SYSTEM

Gut and brain health is of the utmost importance to overall health. To be successful, you need to focus on the signals your body is giving you. For example, if you learn that consuming dairy causes some digestive upset, it is your body's way of telling you to avoid such foods! Keeping a food diary and log could help you identify the latest trends and signs of food consumption. Digestive health is more crucial than many people think.

EATING FOODS TO KEEP YOUR BLOOD SUGAR CONSTANT

Have you ever felt weak or shaky between your meals? Do you have fluctuations in your energy level? Chances are your blood sugar is rising and falling due to your meals. If you eat sugar and white flour, your blood sugar will spike, and you will feel a rush of energy. However, as the body automatically handles sugar, blood sugar will also drop, and you will start to feel hungry and lethargic. Consuming whole foods would give your body carbohydrates, enough protein, and ample amounts of fat. The combination would allow blood sugar to rise even more slowly after meals and stay elevated between meals.

The main thing is that this could easily be customized to fit anyone. For example, keeping a journal about how you feel throughout the day could make the whole process run smoothly.

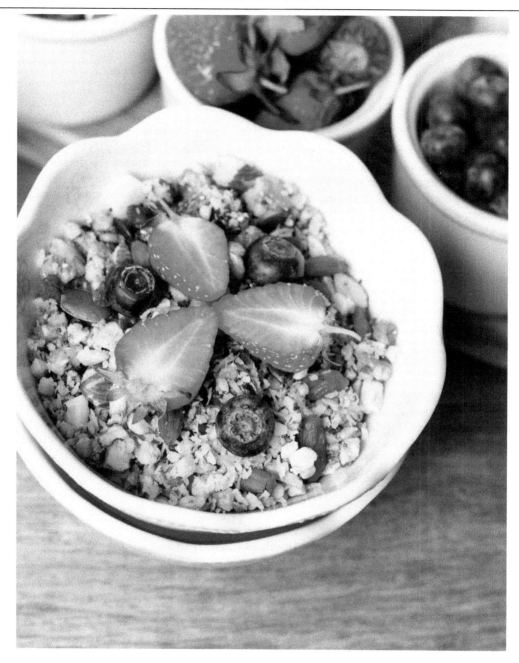

1) **Everyday Blackberry Chia Pudding**

Preparation Time: approx. 45 minutes

Servings: 4

Ingredients:
- ✓ 1 ½ cups coconut milk
- ✓ ½ cup Greek yogurt
- ✓ 4 tsp sugar-free maple syrup
- ✓ 1 tsp vanilla extract
- ✓ 7 tbsp chia seeds

Directions:
- ❖ In a bowl, combine coconut milk, Greek yogurt, sugar-free maple syrup, and vanilla extract until evenly combined. Mix in the chia seeds. Puree half of blackberries in a bowl using a fork and stir in the yogurt mixture

Ingredients:
- ✓ 1 cup fresh blackberries
- ✓ 3 tbsp chopped almonds
- ✓ Mint leaves to garnish

- ❖ . Share the mixture into medium mason jars, cover the lids and refrigerate for 30 minutes to thicken the pudding. Remove the jars, take off the lid, and stir the mixture. Garnish with remaining blackberries, almonds, and some mint leaves.

Nutrition: Calories 309; Net Carbs 6.8g; Fat 26g; Protein 7g

2) **Easy Blueberry Soufflé**

Preparation Time: approx. 35 minutes

Servings: 4

Ingredients:
- ✓ 1 cup frozen blueberries
- ✓ 5 tbsp erythritol
- ✓ 4 egg yolks

Directions:
- ❖ Pour blueberries, 2 tbsp erythritol and 1 tbsp water in a saucepan. Cook until the berries soften and become syrupy, 8-10 minutes. Set aside. Preheat oven to 350 F. In a bowl, beat egg yolks and 1 tbsp of erythritol until thick and pale. In another bowl, whisk egg whites until foamy. Add in remaining erythritol and whisk until soft peak forms, 3-4 minutes.

Ingredients:
- ✓ 3 egg whites
- ✓ 1 tsp olive oil
- ✓ ½ lemon, zested
- ❖ Fold egg white mixture into egg yolk mix. Heat olive oil in a pan over low heat. Add in olive oil and pour in the egg mixture; swirl to spread. Cook for 3 minutes and transfer to the oven; bake for 2-3 minutes or until puffed and set. Plate soufflé and spoon blueberry sauce all over. Garnish with lemon zest.

Nutrition: Calories 99; Net Carbs 2.8g; Fat 5.9g; Protein 5.5g

3) **American Cheddar Biscuits**

Preparation Time: approx. 30 minutes

Servings: 4

Ingredients:
- ✓ 2 ½ cups almond flour
- ✓ 2 tsp baking powder
- ✓ 2 eggs beaten

Directions:
- ❖ Preheat oven to 350 F. Line a baking sheet with parchment paper. In a bowl, mix flour, baking powder, and eggs until smooth. Whisk in the melted butter and cheddar cheese until well combined.

Ingredients:
- ✓ 3 tbsp melted butter
- ✓ ¾ cup grated cheddar cheese

- ❖ Mold 12 balls out of the mixture and arrange on the sheet at 2-inch intervals. Bake for 25 minutes until golden brown. Remove, let cool, and serve.

Nutrition: Calories 355; Net Carbs 1.4g, Fat 28g, Protein 21g

4) Delicious Vanilla Buttermilk Pancakes

Preparation Time: approx. 25 minutes

Servings: 4

Ingredients:

- ✓ ½ cup almond flour
- ✓ ½ tsp baking powder
- ✓ 1 tbsp swerve sugar
- ✓ ½ cup buttermilk
- ✓ 1 lemon, juiced
- ✓ Blueberries to serve

Ingredients:

- ✓ 3 eggs
- ✓ 1 vanilla pod
- ✓ 2 tbsp unsalted butter
- ✓ 2 tbsp olive oil
- ✓ 3 tbsp sugar-free maple syrup
- ✓ Greek yogurt to serve
- ❖ Cook for 4 minutes or until small bubbles appear. Flip and cook for 2 minutes or until set and golden. Repeat cooking until the batter finishes using the remaining butter and olive oil in the same proportions. Plate the pancakes, drizzle with maple syrup, top with a generous dollop of yogurt, and scatter some blueberries on top.

Directions:

- ❖ Into a bowl, mix almond flour, baking powder, and swerve sugar. In a small bowl, whisk buttermilk, lemon juice, and eggs. Combine the mixture with the flour mix until smooth. Cut the vanilla pod open and scrape the beans into the flour mixture. Stir to incorporate evenly. In a skillet, melt a quarter each of the butter and olive oil and spoon in 1 ½ tbsp of the pancake mixture into the pan.

168; Net Carbs 1.6g; Fat 11g; Protein 7g

5) Easy Berry and Mascarpone Bowl

Preparation Time: approx. 10 minutes

Servings: 4

Ingredients:

- ✓ 1 ½ cups blueberries and raspberries
- ✓ 4 cups Greek yogurt
- ✓ 1 tsp liquid stevia

Ingredients:

- ✓ 1 ½ cups mascarpone cheese
- ✓ 1 cup raw pistachios

- ❖ . Divide the mixture into 4 bowls, sprinkle the berries and pistachios on top and serve.

Directions:

- ❖ Mix the yogurt, stevia, and mascarpone in a bowl until evenly combined

Nutrition: Calories 480, Net Carbs 5g, Fat 40g, Protein 20g

6) Special Avocado Halloumi Scones

Preparation Time: approx. 35 minutes

Servings: 4

Ingredients:

- ✓ 1 cup halloumi cheese, grated
- ✓ 2 cups almond flour
- ✓ 3 tsp baking powder
- ✓ ½ cup butter, cold

Ingredients:

- ✓ 1 avocado, pitted and mashed
- ✓ 1 large egg
- ✓ 1/3 cup buttermilk

- ❖ Place on the baking sheet and bake for 25 minutes or until the scones turn a golden color. Let cool before serving.

Directions:

- ❖ Preheat oven to 350 F. Line a baking sheet with parchment paper. In a bowl, combine flour and baking powder. Add in butter and mix. Stir in halloumi cheese, and avocado. Whisk the egg with buttermilk and stir in the halloumi mix. Mold 8-10 scones out to the batter

Nutrition: Calories 432; Net Carbs 2.3g; Fat 42g; Protein 10g

7) Delicious Almond-Berry Pancakes with Sweet Syrup

Preparation Time: approx. 25 minutes

Servings: 4

Ingredients:
- ✓ 1 handful of strawberries and raspberries, mashed
- ✓ 1 handful fresh strawberries and raspberries for topping
- ✓ ½ cup almond flour
- ✓ 1 tsp baking soda
- ✓ A pinch of salt

Ingredients:
- ✓ 1 tbsp swerve sugar
- ✓ A pinch of cinnamon powder
- ✓ 1 egg
- ✓ ½ cup almond milk
- ✓ 2 tsp butter
- ✓ 1 cup Greek yogurt
- ❖ Cook until small bubbles appear, flip, and cook until golden. Transfer to a plate and proceed using up the remaining batter for pancakes. Top pancakes with yogurt and whole berries.

Directions:
- ❖ In a bowl, combine almond flour, baking soda, salt, swerve sugar, and cinnamon. Whisk in mashed berries, egg, and milk until smooth. Melt ½ tsp of butter in a skillet and pour in 1 tbsp of the mixture into the pan

Nutrition: Calories 234; Net Carbs 7.6g; Fat 17g; Protein 9g

8) Special Toast Sticks and Berry Yogurt Bowls

Preparation Time: approx. 15 min + chilling time

Servings: 2

Ingredients:
- ✓ 2 cups Greek yogurt
- ✓ 2 tbsp sugar-free maple syrup
- ✓ ½ cup strawberries, halved
- ✓ ½ cup blueberries
- ✓ ½ cup raspberries
- ✓ 2 eggs

Ingredients:
- ✓ ¼ tsp cinnamon powder
- ✓ ¼ tsp nutmeg powder
- ✓ 2 tbsp almond milk
- ✓ 4 slices zero carb bread
- ✓ 1 ½ tbsp butter
- ✓ 1 tbsp olive oil
- ❖ Dip each strip into the egg mixture and fry in the skillet, flipping once until golden brown on both sides. Transfer to a serving plate and serve warm.

Directions:
- ❖ In a bowl, mix yogurt, maple syrup, and berries. Chill for about 1 hour. In another bowl, whisk eggs, cinnamon, nutmeg, and almond milk. Set aside. Cut each bread slice into four strips. Heat butter and olive oil in a skillet over medium heat.

Nutrition: Calories 207; Net Carbs 7.3g; Fat 14g; Protein 7.7g

9) Easy and Quick Protein Bars

Preparation Time: approx. 5 min + chilling time

Servings: 4

Ingredients:
- ✓ 1 cup almond butter
- ✓ 4 tbsp coconut oil
- ✓ 2 scoops vanilla protein
- ✓ ½ cup sugar-free maple syrup

Ingredients:
- ✓ 4 tbsp unsweetened chocolate chips
- ✓ 1 tsp cinnamon powder
- ✓ 1 tbsp chopped toasted peanuts
- ❖ Spread the mixture onto the sheet and scatter remaining chocolate and peanuts on top. Refrigerate until firm, at least 1 hour. Cut into bars.

Directions:
- ❖ Line a baking sheet with parchment paper. In a bowl, mix almond butter, coconut oil, vanilla protein, maple syrup, 4 tbsp chocolate chips, and cinnamon.

Nutrition: Calories 326; Net Carbs 0.4g, Fat 29g, Protein 0.5g

10) Italian Mascarpone Snapped Amaretti Biscuits

Preparation Time: 25 minutes   Servings: 6

Ingredients:
- ✓ 6 egg whites
- ✓ 1 egg yolk, beaten
- ✓ 1 tsp vanilla bean paste
- ✓ 4 tbsp swerve sugar
- ✓ A pinch of salt
- ✓ ¼ cup ground fragrant almonds

Ingredients:
- ✓ 1 lemon juice
- ✓ 7 tbsp sugar-free amaretto liquor
- ✓ ¼ cup mascarpone cheese
- ✓ ¼ cup butter, room temperature
- ✓ ¾ cup swerve confectioner's sugar

Directions:
- ❖ Preheat oven to 300°F. Line a baking sheet with parchment paper. In a bowl, beat egg whites, salt, and vanilla paste with a hand mixer while you gradually spoon in the swerve sugar until stiff. Add in almonds and fold in the egg yolk, lemon juice, and amaretto liquor. Spoon mixture into a piping bag.
- ❖ Press out 50 mounds on the baking sheet. Bake the biscuits for 15 minutes until golden brown.

- ❖ Transfer to a wire rack to cool. Whisk the mascarpone cheese, butter, and swerve confectioner's sugar with the cleaned electric mixer. Spread a scoop of mascarpone cream onto the case of half of the biscuits and snap with the remaining biscuits. Dust with some swerve confectioner's sugar and serve.

Nutrition: Calories 165, Fat 13g, Net Carbs 3g, Protein 9g

11) Special Turkey Sausage Egg Cups

Preparation Time: 15 minutes   Servings: 4

Ingredients:
- ✓ 2 tsp butter
- ✓ 8 eggs, beaten
- ✓ Salt and black pepper to taste

Ingredients:
- ✓ ½ tsp dried rosemary
- ✓ 1 cup pecorino romano, grated
- ✓ 4 turkey sausages, chopped
- ❖ Divide between greased muffin cups and bake for 4 minutes. Crack an egg into the middle of each cup. Bake for 4 more minutes. Serve cooled.

Directions:
- ❖ Preheat oven to 400°F. Melt butter in a skillet over medium heat. Cook the turkey sausages for 4-5 minutes. In a bowl, mix 4 eggs, sausages, cheese, and seasonings.

Nutrition: Calories 423; Fat: 34.1g, Net Carbs: 2.2g, Protein: 26.5g

12) Easy Cheese Stuffed Avocados

Preparation Time: 20 minutes   Servings: 4

Ingredients:
- ✓ 3 avocados, halved, pitted, skin on
- ✓ ½ cup feta cheese, crumbled
- ✓ ½ cup cheddar cheese, grated

Ingredients:
- ✓ 2 eggs, beaten
- ✓ Salt and black pepper to taste
- ✓ 1 tbsp fresh basil, chopped
- ❖ Split the mixture into the avocado halves. Bake for 15 minutes. Top with basil and serve.

Directions:
- ❖ Preheat oven to 360°F. Lay avocado halves in a baking dish. In a bowl, mix both types of cheeses, pepper, eggs, and salt

Nutrition: Calories 342; Fat: 30.4g, Net Carbs: 7.5g, Protein: 11.1g

13) Special Duo-Cheese Omelet with Pimenta and Basil

Preparation Time: 15 minutes   Servings: 2

Ingredients:

- ✓ 1 tbsp olive oil
- ✓ 4 eggs, beaten
- ✓ Salt and black pepper to taste
- ✓ ¼ tsp paprika

Directions:

- ❖ Warm the olive oil in a pan over medium. Season the eggs with cayenne pepper, salt, paprika, and pepper. Transfer to the pan and ensure they are evenly spread. Cook for 5 minutes

Nutrition: Calories 490; Fat: 44.6g, Net Carbs: 4.5g, Protein: 22.7g

Ingredients:

- ✓ ¼ tsp cayenne pepper
- ✓ ½ cup asiago cheese, shredded
- ✓ ½ cup cheddar cheese, shredded
- ✓ 2 tbsp fresh basil, roughly chopped
- ❖ Top with the asiago and cheddar cheeses. Slice the omelet into two halves. Decorate with fresh basil and serve.

14) Easy and Quick Blue Cheese Omelet

Preparation Time: 15 minutes

Servings: 2

Ingredients:

- ✓ 4 eggs
- ✓ Salt to taste
- ✓ 1 tbsp sesame oil

Directions:

- ❖ In a bowl, beat the eggs with salt. Warm the oil in a pan over medium heat. Add in the eggs and cook as you swirl the eggs around the pan.

Nutrition: Calories 307Calories; Fat: 25g, Net Carbs: 2.5g, Protein: 18.5g

Ingredients:

- ✓ ½ cup blue cheese, crumbled
- ✓ 1 tomato, thinly sliced

- ❖ Cook eggs until set. Top with cheese. Decorate with tomato and serve.

15) Tropical Coconut and Walnut Chia Pudding

Preparation Time: 10 minutes

Servings: 1

Ingredients:

- ✓ ½ tsp vanilla extract
- ✓ ½ cup water
- ✓ 1 tbsp chia seeds
- ✓ 2 tbsp hemp seeds
- ✓ 1 tbsp flaxseed meal

Directions:

- ❖ Put chia seeds, hemp seeds, flaxseed meal, almond meal, stevia, and coconut in a saucepan and pour over the water. Simmer over medium heat, occasionally stirring until creamed and thickened, about 3-4 minutes

Nutrition: Calories Calories 334, Fat: 29g, Net Carbs: 1.5g Protein: 15g

Ingredients:

- ✓ 2 tbsp almond meal
- ✓ 2 tbsp shredded coconut
- ✓ ¼ tsp granulated stevia
- ✓ 1 tbsp walnuts, chopped

- ❖ Stir in vanilla. When it is ready, spoon into a serving bowl, sprinkle with walnuts, and serve.

16) Italian Cheese Ciabatta with Pepperoni

Preparation Time: 30 minutes

Servings: 6

Ingredients:
- ✓ 10 oz cream cheese, melted
- ✓ 2 ½ cups mozzarella, shredded
- ✓ 4 large eggs, beaten
- ✓ 3 tbsp Romano cheese, grated

Directions:
- ❖ In a bowl, combine eggs, mozzarella cheese, cream cheese, baking powder, pork rinds, and Romano cheese. Form into 6 chiabatta shapes

Ingredients:
- ✓ ½ cup pork rinds, crushed
- ✓ 2 tsp baking powder
- ✓ ½ cup tomato puree
- ✓ 12 pepperoni slices
- ❖ Set a pan over medium heat. Cook each ciabatta for 2 minutes per side. Sprinkle tomato puree over each one and top with pepperoni slices to serve.

Nutrition: Calories Calories 464, Fat: 33.6g, Net Carbs: 9.1g, Protein: 31.1g

17) Special Seed Breakfast Loaf

Preparation Time: approx. 55 minutes

Servings: 6

Ingredients:
- ✓ ¾ cup coconut flour
- ✓ 1 cup almond flour
- ✓ 3 tbsp baking powder
- ✓ 2 tbsp psyllium husk powder
- ✓ 2 tbsp desiccated coconut
- ✓ 5 tbsp sesame seeds
- ✓ ¼ cup flaxseed
- ✓ ¼ cup hemp seeds

Directions:
- ❖ Preheat oven to 350 F. In a bowl, mix coconut and almond flours, baking powder, psyllium husk, desiccated coconut, sesame seeds, flaxseed, hemp seeds, ground caraway and poppy seeds, salt, and allspice

Ingredients:
- ✓ 1 tsp ground caraway seeds
- ✓ 1 tbsp poppy seeds
- ✓ 1 tsp salt
- ✓ 1 tsp allspice
- ✓ 6 eggs
- ✓ 1 cup cream cheese, softened
- ✓ ¾ cup heavy cream
- ✓ 4 tbsp sesame oil
- ❖ In another bowl, whisk eggs, cream cheese, heavy cream, and sesame oil. Pour the mixture into the dry ingredients and combine both into a smooth dough. Pour the dough in a greased loaf pan. Bake for 45 minutes. Remove onto a rack and let cool.

Nutrition: Calories 584; Net Carbs 7.4g; Fat 50g; Protein 23g

18) **Easy Blueberry Chia Pudding**

Preparation Time: approx. 10 min + chilling time

Servings: 2

Ingredients:
- ✓ ¾ cup coconut milk
- ✓ ½ tsp vanilla extract
- ✓ ½ cup blueberries

Directions:
- ❖ In a blender, pour coconut milk, vanilla extract, and half of the blueberries. Process the ingredients in high speed until the blueberries have incorporated into the liquid

Ingredients:
- ✓ 2 tbsp chia seeds
- ✓ 1 tbsp chopped walnuts

- ❖ . Mix in chia seeds. Share the mixture into 2 breakfast jars, cover, and refrigerate for 4 hours to allow it to gel. Garnish with the remaining blueberries and walnuts. Serve.

Nutrition: Calories 301; Net Carbs 6g; Fat 23g; Protein 9g

19) **Easy Creamy Sesame Bread**

Preparation Time: approx. 40 minutes

Servings: 6

Ingredients:
- ✓ 4 tbsp flax seed powder
- ✓ 1 cup cream cheese
- ✓ 5 tbsp sesame oil
- ✓ 1 cup coconut flour

Directions:
- ❖ In a bowl, mix flax seed powder with 1 ½ cups water until smoothly combined and set aside to soak for 5 minutes. Preheat oven to 400 F. When the flax egg is ready, beat in cream cheese and 4 tbsp sesame oil until mixed. Whisk in coconut flour, psyllium husk powder, salt, and baking powder until adequately blended

Ingredients:
- ✓ 2 tbsp psyllium husk powder
- ✓ 1 tsp salt
- ✓ 1 tsp baking powder
- ✓ 1 tbsp sesame seeds
- ❖ Spread the dough in a greased baking tray. Allow to stand for 5 minutes and then brush with remaining sesame oil. Sprinkle with sesame seeds and bake the dough for 30 minutes. Slice and serve.

Nutrition: Calories 285; Net Carbs 1g; Fat 26g; Protein 8g

20) **Special Bulletproof Coffee**

Preparation Time: approx. 3 minutes

Servings: 2

Ingredients:
- ✓ 2 ½ heaping tbsp ground bulletproof coffee beans
- ✓ 1 tbsp coconut oil

Directions:
- ❖ Using a coffee maker, brew one cup of coffee with the ground coffee beans and 1 cup of water. Transfer the coffee to a blender and add the coconut oil and butter

Ingredients:
- ✓ 2 tbsp unsalted butter

- ❖ Blend the mixture until frothy and smooth.

Nutrition: Calories 336; Net Carbs 0g; Fat 36g; Protein 2g

21) Easy Breakfast Naan Bread

Preparation Time: approx. 25 minutes

Servings: 6

Ingredients:
- ¾ cup almond flour
- 2 tbsp psyllium husk powder
- 1 tsp salt
- ½ tsp baking powder

Ingredients:
- ¼ cup olive oil
- 2 cups boiling water
- 8 oz butter
- 2 garlic cloves, minced
- . Melt half of the butter in a frying pan over medium heat and fry the naan on both sides to have a golden color. Transfer to a plate and keep warm. Add the remaining butter to the pan and sauté garlic until fragrant, about 1 minute. Pour the garlic butter into a bowl and serve as a dip along with the naan.

Directions:
- In a bowl, mix almond flour, psyllium husk powder, ½ tsp of salt, and baking powder. Mix in olive oil and boiling water to combine the ingredients like a thick porridge. Stir and allow the dough rise for 5 minutes. Divide the dough into 6 pieces and mold into balls. Place the balls on a parchment paper and flatten

Nutrition: Calories 224; Net Carbs 3g; Fat 19g; Protein 4g

22) Italian-style Fontina Cheese and Chorizo Waffles

Preparation Time: 30 minutes

Servings: 6

Ingredients:
- 6 eggs
- 2 tbsp butter, melted
- 1 cup almond flour

Ingredients:
- Salt and black pepper to taste
- 3 chorizo sausages, cooked, chopped
- 1 cup fontina cheese, shredded
- Preheat the waffle iron and grease it with cooking spray. Pour in the egg mixture and cook for 5 minutes until golden brown. Serve hot.

Directions:
- In a shallow bowl, beat the eggs with salt and pepper. Add in the almond milk, butter, fontina cheese, and sausages and stir to combine. Let it sit for 15-20 minutes

Nutrition: Calories 316; Fat: 25g, Net Carbs: 1.5g, Protein: 20.2g

23) Tropical Coconut Porridge with Strawberries

Preparation Time: approx. 12 minutes

Servings: 2

Ingredients:
- Flax egg: 1 tbsp flax seed powder + 3 tbsp water
- 1 oz olive oil
- 1 tbsp coconut flour

Ingredients:
- 1 pinch ground chia seeds
- 5 tbsp coconut cream
- 1 pinch salt
- Strawberries to serve
- Cook, while stirring continuously until the desired consistency is achieved. Top with strawberries.

Directions:
- For flax egg, in a bowl, mix flax seed powder with water, and let soak for 5 minutes. Place a saucepan over low heat and pour in olive oil, flax egg, flour, chia, coconut cream, and salt.

Nutrition: Calories 521; Net Carbs 4g; Fat 49g; Protein 10g

24) **Original Mexican Tofu Scramble**

Preparation Time: approx. 45 minutes

Servings: 4

Ingredients:
- ✓ 8 oz tofu, scrambled
- ✓ 2 tbsp butter
- ✓ 1 green bell pepper, chopped
- ✓ 1 tomato, finely chopped

Directions:
- ❖ Melt butter in a skillet over medium heat. Fry the tofu until golden brown, stirring occasionally, about 5 minutes.

Ingredients:
- ✓ 2 tbsp chopped scallions
- ✓ Salt and black pepper to taste
- ✓ 1 tsp Mexican chili powder
- ✓ 3 oz grated Parmesan cheese
- ❖ . Stir in bell pepper, tomato, scallions, and cook until the vegetables are soft, 4 minutes. Season with salt, pepper, chili powder and stir in Parmesan cheese, about 2 minutes. Spoon the scramble into a serving platter and serve warm.

Nutrition: Calories254; Net Carbs 3g; Fat 19g; Protein 16g

25) **Special No-Bread Avocado Sandwiches**

Preparation Time: approx. 10 minutes

Servings: 2

Ingredients:
- ✓ 1 avocado, sliced
- ✓ 1 large red tomato, sliced
- ✓ 4 little gem lettuce leaves

Directions:
- ❖ Arrange the lettuce on a flat serving plate. Smear each leave with butter and arrange tofu slices on the leaves

Ingredients:
- ✓ ½ oz butter, softened
- ✓ 4 tofu slices
- ✓ 1 tsp chopped parsley
- ❖ Top with the avocado and tomato slices. Garnish the sandwiches with parsley and serve.

Nutrition: Calories 385; Net Carbs 4g; Fat 32g; Protein 12g

26) **Paleo Eggs and Crabmeat with Creme Fraiche Salsa**

Preparation Time: 15 minutes

Servings: 3

Ingredients:
- ✓ 1 tbsp olive oil
- ✓ 6 eggs, whisked
- ✓ 1 (6 oz) can crabmeat, flaked
- ✓ Salsa
- ✓ ¾ cup crème fraiche

Directions:
- ❖ Warm the olive oil a pan over medium heat. Add in the eggs and scramble them. Stir in crabmeat and season with salt and pepper. Cook until cooked thoroughly. In a dish, combine all salsa ingredients

Ingredients:
- ✓ ½ cup scallions, chopped
- ✓ ½ tsp garlic powder
- ✓ Salt and black pepper to taste
- ✓ ½ tsp fresh dill, chopped

- ❖ . Split the egg/crabmeat mixture among serving plates. Serve alongside the scallions and salsa to the side.

Nutrition: Calories 334; Fat: 26.2g, Net Carbs: 4.4g, Protein: 21.1g

27) **Easy Cheese and Aioli Eggs**

Preparation Time: 20 minutes

Ingredients:

- ✓ 4 eggs, hard-boiled and chopped
- ✓ 14 oz tuna in brine, drained
- ✓ ¼ lettuce head, torn into pieces
- ✓ 2 green onions, finely chopped
- ✓ ½ cup feta cheese, crumbled

Directions:

- ❖ Set the eggs in a serving bowl. Place in tuna, onion, feta cheese, lettuce, and sour cream. In a bowl, mix the mayonnaise, lemon juice, and garlic

Nutrition: Calories 355; Fat 22.5g, Net Carbs 1.8g, Protein 29.5g

Servings: 4

Ingredients:

- ✓ ⅓ cup sour cream
- ✓ Aioli
- ✓ 1 cup mayonnaise
- ✓ 2 cloves garlic, minced
- ✓ 1 tbsp lemon juice
- ✓ Salt and black pepper to taste
- ❖ Season with salt and pepper. Pour the aioli into the serving bowl and stir to incorporate everything. Serve with pickles.

28) **Special Kielbasa and Roquefort Waffles**

Preparation Time: 20 minutes

Ingredients:

- ✓ ½ tsp parsley, chopped
- ✓ ½ tsp chili pepper flakes
- ✓ 4 eggs

Directions:

- ❖ In a bowl, combine all ingredients except chives. Preheat the waffle iron. Pour in some batter and close the lid

Nutrition: Calories 470; Fat: 40.3g, Net Carbs: 2.9g, Protein: 24.4g

Servings: 2

Ingredients:

- ✓ ½ cup Roquefort cheese, crumbled
- ✓ 4 slices kielbasa, chopped
- ✓ 2 tbsp fresh chives, chopped
- ❖ Cook for 5 minutes until golden brown. Repeat with the rest of the batter. Decorate with chives.

29) **Rich Baked Quail Eggs in Avocados**

Preparation Time: 15 minutes

Ingredients:

- ✓ 2 large avocados, halved and pitted
- ✓ 4 small eggs

Directions:

- ❖ Preheat oven to 400°F. Crack the quail eggs into the avocado halves and place them on a greased baking sheet.

Nutrition: Calories 234, Fat 19.1g, Net Carbs 2.2g, Protein 8.2g

Servings: 4

Ingredients:

- ✓ Salt and black pepper to taste

- ❖ Bake the filled avocados in the oven for 8-10 minutes until eggs are cooked. Season and serve.

LUNCH & DINNER

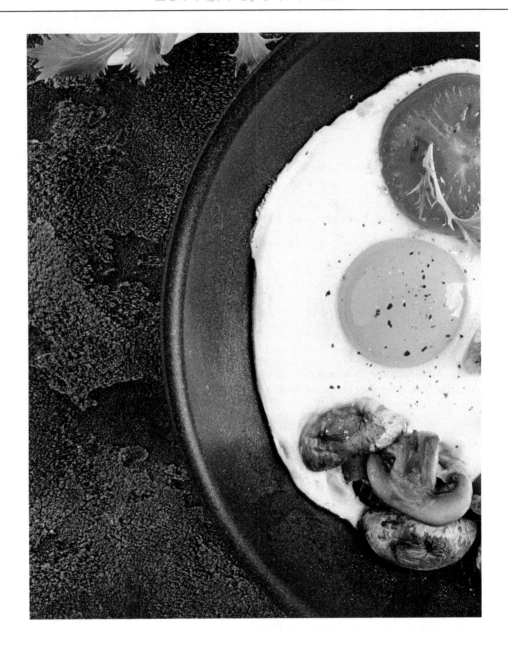

30) **Special Healthy Paleo Oxtail Stew**

Preparation Time: 1 hour 15 minutes

Servings: 8

Ingredients:

- ✓ 4 and ½ lb. oxtail, cut into medium chunks
- ✓ A drizzle of extra virgin olive oil
- ✓ 1 tbsp. extra virgin olive oil
- ✓ 2 leeks, chopped
- ✓ 4 carrots, chopped
- ✓ 2 celery sticks, chopped
- ✓ 4 thyme springs, chopped
- ✓ 4 rosemary springs, chopped
- ✓ 4 cloves

Ingredients:

- ✓ 4 bay leaves
- ✓ Salt and black pepper to taste
- ✓ 2 tbsp. flour
- ✓ 28 oz. can plum tomatoes, chopped
- ✓ 9 oz. red wine
- ✓ 1 quart beef stock
- ✓ Worcestershire sauce to taste

Directions:

- ❖ In a roasting pan, mix oxtail with salt and pepper and a drizzle of oil.
- ❖ Toss to coat, introduce in the oven at 425 degrees and bake for 20 minutes.
- ❖ Heat up a pot with one tbsp oil over medium heat, add leeks, celery, and carrots, stir and cook for 4 minutes.
- ❖ Add thyme, rosemary and bay leaves, stir and cook everything for 20 minutes.
- ❖ Take oxtail out of the oven and leave aside for a few moments.
- ❖ Add flour and cloves to veggies and stir.

- ❖ Also add tomatoes, wine, oxtail and its juices and stock, stir, increase heat to high and bring to a boil.
- ❖ Introduce pot in the oven at 325 degrees and bake for 5 hours.
- ❖ Take stew out of the oven, leave aside for 10 minutes, take oxtail out of the pot and discard bones.
- ❖ Return meat to pot, add more salt and pepper to the taste and some Worcestershire sauce, stir, transfer to plates and serve.
- ❖ Enjoy!

Nutrition: Calories 123 | Fat: 38g | Carbs: 12g |Protein: 28g | Fiber: 2.6g | Sugar: 0g

31) **Easy Paleo Eggplant Stew**

Preparation Time: 40 minutes

Servings:3

Ingredients:

- ✓ 1 eggplant, chopped
- ✓ 1 yellow onion, chopped
- ✓ 2 tomatoes, chopped
- ✓ 1 tsp cumin powder

Ingredients:

- ✓ Salt and black pepper to taste
- ✓ 1 cup tomato paste
- ✓ A pinch of cayenne pepper
- ✓ ½ cup water
- ❖ Take stew off heat, add more salt and pepper if needed, transfer to plates and serve.
- ❖ Enjoy!

Directions:

- ❖ Heat up a pan over medium-high heat, add water, tomato paste, salt and pepper, cayenne and cumin and stir well.
- ❖ Add the eggplant, tomato, and onion, stir, bring to a boil, reduce heat to medium and cook for 30 minutes.

Nutrition: Calories 82 | Fat: 0g | Carbs: 16g | Protein: 5g | Fiber: 1g | Sugar: 0.5g

32) Salmon with sour cream and parmesan cheese

Preparation Time: 25 minutes

Servings: 4

Ingredients:
- ✓ 1 cup sour cream
- ✓ 1 tbsp fresh dill, chopped
- ✓ ½ lemon, peeled and squeezed

Directions:
- ❖ Preheat oven to 400°F. In a bowl, mix the sour cream, dill, lemon zest, juice, salt and pepper. Season the fish with salt and black pepper, pour the lemon juice over both sides of the fish and arrange on a lined baking sheet.

Ingredients:
- ✓ Pink salt and black pepper to taste
- ✓ 4 slices of salmon
- ✓ ½ cup Parmesan cheese, grated
- ❖ Spread the sour cream mixture over each fish and sprinkle with Parmesan cheese.
- ❖ Bake the fish for 15 minutes and then bake the top for 2 minutes with a careful eye for a nice brown color. Plate the fish and serve with buttered green beans.

Nutrition: Calories 288, Fat 23.4g, Net Carbs 1.2g, Protein 16.2g

33) Salmon with herbs in creamy sauce

Preparation Time: 15 minutes

Servings: 2

Ingredients:
- ✓ 2 salmon fillets
- ✓ 1 tsp dried tarragon
- ✓ 1 tsp dried dill

Directions:
- ❖ Season the salmon with some of the dill and tarragon. Heat the butter in a skillet over medium heat. Add the salmon and cook for 4 minutes on both sides. Set aside. In the same skillet, add the remaining dill and tarragon.

Ingredients:
- ✓ 3 tbsp butter
- ✓ ¼ cup heavy cream
- ✓ Salt and black pepper to taste
- ❖ Cook for 30 seconds to infuse the flavors. Whisk in the heavy cream, season with salt and black pepper and cook for 2-3 minutes. Serve the salmon topped with the sauce.

Nutrition: Calories 468, Fat: 40g, Net Carbs: 1.5g, Protein: 22g

34) Salmon in pistachio crust with asparagus

Preparation Time: 35 minutes

Servings: 4

Ingredients:
- ✓ 4 salmon fillets
- ✓ Salt and black pepper to taste
- ✓ 1 tbsp Dijon mustard
- ✓ 2 tbsp chopped pork rind

Directions:
- ❖ Preheat oven to 370°F. In a small bowl, combine pork rind, pistachios and 1 tbsp olive oil; stir with a fork to combine. Brush salmon with Dijon mustard and season with salt and pepper.

Ingredients:
- ✓ ½ cup chopped pistachios
- ✓ 2 tbsp chopped fresh dill
- ✓ 2 tbsp olive oil
- ✓ 1 lemon, cut into wedges
- ✓ 1 pound asparagus
- ❖ Press the pistachio mixture over the salmon to form a crust. Coat the asparagus with the remaining olive oil and season with salt and pepper in a bowl. Lay the salmon on a greased baking sheet. Arrange asparagus around salmon and bake for 15-20 minutes until salmon is flaky to the touch. Top with chopped dill and serve with lemon wedges on the side.

Nutrition: Calories 474, Fat: 31, Net Carbohydrates: 3.8g, Protein: 44.4g

35) **Steamed salmon with creamy cucumber sauce**

Preparation Time: 30 minutes   **Servings: 4**

Ingredients:

- ✓ 4 salmon fillets with skin on
- ✓ 10 ounces of broccoli florets
- ✓ 2 tbsp olive oil
- ✓ 1 cucumber, diced

Directions:

- ❖ Combine the cucumber, crème fraiche, fresh dill and lemon juice in a bowl. Season with salt and mix thoroughly. Cover and refrigerate to chill until ready to use.
- ❖ Fill a large pot halfway with water and place in a steamer basket; bring to a boil. Add broccoli florets and season with salt.

Ingredients:

- ✓ 1 cup creme fraiche
- ✓ ¼ tbsp lemon juice
- ✓ Salt and black pepper to taste
- ✓ 2 tbsp fresh dill
- ❖ Steam the broccoli for 6 minutes, until tender-crisp but still a vibrant green. Transfer to a bowl and drizzle with olive oil; cover with aluminum foil to maintain heat.
- ❖ Place the salmon in the basket, skin side down, and sprinkle with salt and pepper. Cook for 8-10 minutes until the fish flakes easily. Serve the salmon topped with the cucumber sauce and broccoli on the side.

Nutrition: Calories 458, Fat 30.4g, Net Carbohydrates 2.6g, Protein 39.1g

36) **Chicken Thighs with Tasty Butternut Squash**

Preparation Time: 30 minutes   **Servings: 4**

Ingredients:

- ✓ 6 chicken thighs, boneless and skinless
- ✓ ½ pound of bacon, chopped
- ✓ 2 tbsp coconut oil

Directions:

- ❖ Heat a skillet over medium heat, add bacon, cook until crispy, drain on paper towels, transfer to a plate, crumble and set aside for now.
- ❖ Heat the same skillet over medium heat, add squash, salt and pepper to taste, stir, cook until soft, transfer to a plate and also set aside.

Ingredients:

- ✓ Handful of sage, chopped
- ✓ Salt and black pepper to taste
- ✓ 3 cups butternut squash, cubed
- ❖ Reheat the skillet with the coconut oil over medium-high heat, add the chicken, salt and pepper and cook for 10 minutes, turning often.
- ❖ Remove skillet from heat, add squash, introduce into 425 degree oven and cook for 15 minutes.
- ❖ Divide chicken and knob of butter among plates, top with sage and bacon and serve.
- ❖ Enjoy!

Nutrition: Calories 241 | Fat: 11g | Carbohydrates: 17g | Protein: 16g | Fiber: 2.5g | Sugar: 0g

37) **Paleo Turkey Casserole**

Preparation Time: 30 minutes

Servings: 4

Ingredients:

- ✓ 1 sweet potato, chopped
- ✓ 1 pound turkey meat, ground
- ✓ 1 eggplant, thinly sliced
- ✓ 1 yellow onion, finely chopped
- ✓ 1 tbsp garlic, finely chopped
- ✓ Salt and black pepper to taste
- ✓ ¼ tsp chili powder
- ✓ ¼ tsp cumin
- ✓ 15 ounces canned tomatoes, chopped and drained
- ✓ 8 ounces of tomato paste

Ingredients:

- ✓ Cooking spray
- ✓ ½ tsp tarragon flakes
- ✓ ⅛ tsp cardamom, ground
- ✓ ⅛ tsp oregano
- ✓ For the sauce:
- ✓ 1 tbsp almond flour
- ✓ 1 cup almond milk
- ✓ 1 ½ tbsp extra virgin olive oil
- ✓ 1 tbsp coconut flour

Directions:

- ❖ Heat a skillet over medium-high heat, add turkey meat, onion and garlic, stir and cook until meat turns brown.
- ❖ Add tomatoes, tomato paste and sweet potatoes, stir and cook for 5 minutes.
- ❖ Add salt, pepper to taste, chili powder, cumin, oregano, tarragon flakes and cardamom, mix well and cook for 2 minutes.
- ❖ Evenly distribute turkey mix, place dish in 350 degree oven and bake for 15 minutes.

- ❖ Meanwhile, heat a saucepan over medium-high heat, add olive oil, almond flour and coconut one, stir well 1 minute, reduce heat, add almond milk and stir well.
- ❖ Cook this for 10 minutes.
- ❖ Introduce again in the oven and bake for 45 minutes.
- ❖ Remove casserole from oven, set aside a few moments to cool, slice and divide among plates and serve.
- ❖ Enjoy!

Nutrition: Calories 278 | Fat: 2.6g | Carbohydrates: 29g| Protein: 28.5g | Fiber: 6.7g | Sugar: 0g

38) **Special Paleo Chicken and Vegetables Stir Fry**

Preparation Time: 30 minutes

Servings: 4

Ingredients:

- ✓ 1 red bell bell pepper, chopped
- ✓ 1 zucchini, chopped
- ✓ 1 yellow onion, finely chopped
- ✓ 1 head of broccoli, florets separated
- ✓ 4 chicken breasts, skinless, boned and trimmed
- ✓ Salt and black pepper to taste
- ✓ 1 tbsp coconut oil
- ✓ ¼ tsp ginger, grated

Ingredients:

For the sauce:
- ✓ ¼ cup chicken broth
- ✓ 2 cloves garlic, finely chopped
- ✓ 3 tbsp coconut aminos
- ✓ ½ cup orange juice
- ✓ 1 tbsp orange zest
- ✓ 1 tbsp Sriracha sauce
- ✓ A pinch of red pepper flakes
- ❖ Add salt, pepper, the orange sauce you made, stir, bring to a boil, add chicken, reduce heat and simmer for 8 minutes.
- ❖ Divide among plates and serve hot.
- ❖ Enjoy!

Directions:

- ❖ In a bowl, mix broth with orange juice, zest, amino, ginger, garlic, pepper flakes and Sriracha sauce and mix well.
- ❖ Heat a skillet with oil over medium heat, add chicken, cook for 8 minutes and transfer to a plate.
- ❖ Heat the same skillet over medium heat, add bell bell pepper, broccoli florets, onion and zucchini, stir and cook for 4-5 minutes.

Nutrition: Calories 320 | Fat: 13g | Carbohydrates: 17g | Protein: 45g | Fiber: 3.7g | Sugar: 0g

39) Paleo Stuffed Quail

Preparation Time: 1 hour and 15 minutes

Servings: 4

Ingredients:

- ✓ 8 slices of bacon
- ✓ 4 quails
- ✓ 1 apple, chopped
- ✓ 1 pound of grapes
- ✓ 1 tbsp chopped rosemary
- ✓ ½ cup cranberries, chopped

Directions:

- ❖ Pat quail dry, season with salt and pepper and set aside for now.
- ❖ In a bowl, mix blueberries with chopped rosemary, apple, olive oil, garlic, salt and pepper to taste and mix well.
- ❖ Fill quail with this combination, wrap each with two slices of bacon and tie with kitchen twine.

Ingredients:

- ✓ 2 tbsp extra virgin olive oil
- ✓ 2 cloves garlic, minced
- ✓ 4 springs of rosemary
- ✓ ½ cup chicken broth
- ✓ Salt and black pepper to taste

- ❖ Spread half of the grapes in an oven dish, mash gently with a fork, arrange the quail on top, scatter the rest of the grapes and pour in the chicken broth at the end.
- ❖ Introduce the whole in the oven at 425 degrees and bake for 1 hour.
- ❖ Divide among plates and serve with roasted grapes on the side.
- ❖ Enjoy!

Nutrition: Calories 260 | Fat: 18g | Carbohydrates: 22g | Protein: 29g | Fiber: 3g | Sugar: 0g

40) Paleo dish of roast duck

Preparation Time 2 hours 10 minutes

Servings: 4

Ingredients:

- ✓ 2 tbsp ground allspice
- ✓ 4 duck legs
- ✓ 4 springs of thyme
- ✓ 1 lemon, sliced

Directions:

- ❖ Arrange half of the lemon and orange slices in the bottom of an oven dish, place the duck legs, top with the rest of the orange and lemon slices and thyme springs.

Ingredients:

- ✓ 1 orange, sliced
- ✓ 1 cup chicken stock
- ✓ Salt and black pepper to taste
- ✓ ½ cup orange juice
- ❖ Add chicken broth, orange juice, sprinkle with allspice, place in 350 degree F oven and bake for 2 hours.
- ❖ Divide among plates and serve hot.
- ❖ Enjoy!

Nutrition: Calories 255 | Fat: 17g | Carbohydrates: 6g | Protein: 33g | Fiber: 1g | Sugar: 0g

41) **Chicken Thighs with Tasty Butternut Squash**

Preparation Time: 30 minutes   **Servings: 4**

Ingredients:
- ✓ 6 chicken thighs, boneless and skinless
- ✓ ½ pound of bacon, chopped
- ✓ 2 tbsp coconut oil

Directions:
- ❖ Heat a skillet over medium heat, add bacon, cook until crispy, drain on paper towels, transfer to a plate, crumble and set aside for now.
- ❖ Heat the same skillet over medium heat, add squash, salt and pepper to taste, stir, cook until soft, transfer to a plate and also set aside.

Ingredients:
- ✓ Handful of sage, chopped
- ✓ Salt and black pepper to taste
- ✓ 3 cups butternut squash, cubed
- ❖ Reheat the skillet with the coconut oil over medium-high heat, add the chicken, salt and pepper and cook for 10 minutes, turning often.
- ❖ Remove skillet from heat, add squash, introduce into 425 degree oven and cook for 15 minutes.
- ❖ Divide chicken and knob of butter among plates, top with sage and bacon and serve.
- ❖ Enjoy!

Nutrition: Calories 241 | Fat: 11g | Carbohydrates: 17g | Protein: 16g | Fiber: 2.5g | Sugar: 0g

42) **Paleo Turkey Casserole**

Preparation Time: 30 minutes   **Servings: 4**

Ingredients:
- ✓ 1 sweet potato, chopped
- ✓ 1 pound turkey meat, ground
- ✓ 1 eggplant, thinly sliced
- ✓ 1 yellow onion, finely chopped
- ✓ 1 tbsp garlic, finely chopped
- ✓ Salt and black pepper to taste
- ✓ ¼ tsp chili powder
- ✓ ¼ tsp cumin
- ✓ 15 ounces canned tomatoes, chopped and drained
- ✓ 8 ounces of tomato paste

Directions:
- ❖ Heat a skillet over medium-high heat, add turkey meat, onion and garlic, stir and cook until meat turns brown.
- ❖ Add tomatoes, tomato paste and sweet potatoes, stir and cook for 5 minutes.
- ❖ Add salt, pepper to taste, chili powder, cumin, oregano, tarragon flakes and cardamom, mix well and cook for 2 minutes.
- ❖ Evenly distribute turkey mix, place dish in 350 degree oven and bake for 15 minutes.

Ingredients:
- ✓ Cooking spray
- ✓ ½ tsp tarragon flakes
- ✓ ⅛ tsp cardamom, ground
- ✓ ⅛ tsp oregano
- ✓ For the sauce:
- ✓ 1 tbsp almond flour
- ✓ 1 cup almond milk
- ✓ 1 ½ tbsp extra virgin olive oil
- ✓ 1 tbsp coconut flour

- ❖ Meanwhile, heat a saucepan over medium-high heat, add olive oil, almond flour and coconut one, stir well 1 minute, reduce heat, add almond milk and stir well.
- ❖ Cook this for 10 minutes.
- ❖ Introduce again in the oven and bake for 45 minutes.
- ❖ Remove casserole from oven, set aside a few moments to cool, slice and divide among plates and serve.
- ❖ Enjoy!

Nutrition: Calories 278 | Fat: 2.6g | Carbohydrates: 29g| Protein: 28.5g | Fiber: 6.7g | Sugar: 0g

43) **Salmon with herbs in creamy sauce**

Preparation Time: 15 minutes

Ingredients:
- ✓ 2 salmon fillets
- ✓ 1 tsp dried tarragon
- ✓ 1 tsp dried dill

Directions:
- ❖ Season the salmon with some of the dill and tarragon. Heat the butter in a skillet over medium heat. Add the salmon and cook for 4 minutes on both sides. Set aside. In the same skillet, add the remaining dill and tarragon.

Servings: 2

Ingredients:
- ✓ 3 tbsp butter
- ✓ ¼ cup heavy cream
- ✓ Salt and black pepper to taste
- ❖ Cook for 30 seconds to infuse the flavors. Whisk in the heavy cream, season with salt and black pepper and cook for 2-3 minutes. Serve the salmon topped with the sauce.

Nutrition: Calories 468, Fat: 40g, Net Carbs: 1.5g, Protein: 22g

44) **Salmon in pistachio crust with asparagus**

Preparation Time: 35 minutes

Ingredients:
- ✓ 4 salmon fillets
- ✓ Salt and black pepper to taste
- ✓ 1 tbsp Dijon mustard
- ✓ 2 tbsp chopped pork rind

Directions:
- ❖ Preheat oven to 370°F. In a small bowl, combine pork rind, pistachios and 1 tbsp olive oil; stir with a fork to combine. Brush salmon with Dijon mustard and season with salt and pepper.

Servings: 4

Ingredients:
- ✓ ½ cup chopped pistachios
- ✓ 2 tbsp chopped fresh dill
- ✓ 2 tbsp olive oil
- ✓ 1 lemon, cut into wedges
- ✓ 1 pound asparagus
- ❖ Press the pistachio mixture over the salmon to form a crust. Coat the asparagus with the remaining olive oil and season with salt and pepper in a bowl. Lay the salmon on a greased baking sheet. Arrange asparagus around salmon and bake for 15-20 minutes until salmon is flaky to the touch. Top with chopped dill and serve with lemon wedges on the side.

Nutrition: Calories 474, Fat: 31, Net Carbohydrates: 3.8g, Protein: 44.4g

45) Steamed salmon with creamy cucumber sauce

Preparation Time: 30 minutes

Servings: 4

Ingredients:

- ✓ 4 salmon fillets with skin on
- ✓ 10 ounces of broccoli florets
- ✓ 2 tbsp olive oil
- ✓ 1 cucumber, diced

Directions:

- ❖ Combine the cucumber, crème fraiche, fresh dill and lemon juice in a bowl. Season with salt and mix thoroughly. Cover and refrigerate to chill until ready to use.
- ❖ Fill a large pot halfway with water and place in a steamer basket; bring to a boil. Add broccoli florets and season with salt.

Ingredients:

- ✓ 1 cup creme fraiche
- ✓ ¼ tbsp lemon juice
- ✓ Salt and black pepper to taste
- ✓ 2 tbsp fresh dill
- ❖ Steam the broccoli for 6 minutes, until tender-crisp but still a vibrant green. Transfer to a bowl and drizzle with olive oil; cover with aluminum foil to maintain heat.
- ❖ Place the salmon in the basket, skin side down, and sprinkle with salt and pepper. Cook for 8-10 minutes until the fish flakes easily. Serve the salmon topped with the cucumber sauce and broccoli on the side.

Nutrition: Calories 458, Fat 30.4g, Net Carbohydrates 2.6g, Protein 39.1g

46) Special Healthy Paleo Oxtail Stew

Preparation Time: 1 hour 15 minutes

Servings: 8

Ingredients:

- ✓ 4 and ½ lb. oxtail, cut into medium chunks
- ✓ A drizzle of extra virgin olive oil
- ✓ 1 tbsp. extra virgin olive oil
- ✓ 2 leeks, chopped
- ✓ 4 carrots, chopped
- ✓ 2 celery sticks, chopped
- ✓ 4 thyme springs, chopped
- ✓ 4 rosemary springs, chopped
- ✓ 4 cloves

Directions:

- ❖ In a roasting pan, mix oxtail with salt and pepper and a drizzle of oil.
- ❖ Toss to coat, introduce in the oven at 425 degrees and bake for 20 minutes.
- ❖ Heat up a pot with one tbsp oil over medium heat, add leeks, celery, and carrots, stir and cook for 4 minutes.
- ❖ Add thyme, rosemary and bay leaves, stir and cook everything for 20 minutes.
- ❖ Take oxtail out of the oven and leave aside for a few moments.
- ❖ Add flour and cloves to veggies and stir.

Ingredients:

- ✓ 4 bay leaves
- ✓ Salt and black pepper to taste
- ✓ 2 tbsp. flour
- ✓ 28 oz. can plum tomatoes, chopped
- ✓ 9 oz. red wine
- ✓ 1 quart beef stock
- ✓ Worcestershire sauce to taste

- ❖ Also add tomatoes, wine, oxtail and its juices and stock, stir, increase heat to high and bring to a boil.
- ❖ Introduce pot in the oven at 325 degrees and bake for 5 hours.
- ❖ Take stew out of the oven, leave aside for 10 minutes, take oxtail out of the pot and discard bones.
- ❖ Return meat to pot, add more salt and pepper to the taste and some Worcestershire sauce, stir, transfer to plates and serve.
- ❖ Enjoy!

Nutrition: Calories 123 | Fat: 38g | Carbs: 12g | Protein: 28g | Fiber: 2.6g | Sugar: 0g

47) **Easy Paleo Eggplant Stew**

Preparation Time: 40 minutes

Servings:3

Ingredients:

- ✓ 1 eggplant, chopped
- ✓ 1 yellow onion, chopped
- ✓ 2 tomatoes, chopped
- ✓ 1 tsp cumin powder

Directions:

- ❖ Heat up a pan over medium-high heat, add water, tomato paste, salt and pepper, cayenne and cumin and stir well.
- ❖ Add the eggplant, tomato, and onion, stir, bring to a boil, reduce heat to medium and cook for 30 minutes.

Ingredients:

- ✓ Salt and black pepper to taste
- ✓ 1 cup tomato paste
- ✓ A pinch of cayenne pepper
- ✓ ½ cup water
- ❖ Take stew off heat, add more salt and pepper if needed, transfer to plates and serve.
- ❖ Enjoy!

Nutrition: Calories 82 | Fat: 0g | Carbs: 16g | Protein: 5g | Fiber: 1g | Sugar: 0.5g

48) **Salmon with sour cream and parmesan cheese**

Preparation Time: 25 minutes

Servings: 4

Ingredients:

- ✓ 1 cup sour cream
- ✓ 1 tbsp fresh dill, chopped
- ✓ ½ lemon, peeled and squeezed

Directions:

- ❖ Preheat oven to 400°F. In a bowl, mix the sour cream, dill, lemon zest, juice, salt and pepper. Season the fish with salt and black pepper, pour the lemon juice over both sides of the fish and arrange on a lined baking sheet.

Ingredients:

- ✓ Pink salt and black pepper to taste
- ✓ 4 slices of salmon
- ✓ ½ cup Parmesan cheese, grated
- ❖ Spread the sour cream mixture over each fish and sprinkle with Parmesan cheese.
- ❖ Bake the fish for 15 minutes and then bake the top for 2 minutes with a careful eye for a nice brown color. Plate the fish and serve with buttered green beans.

Nutrition: Calories 288, Fat 23.4g, Net Carbs 1.2g, Protein 16.2g

49) **Olives and Avocado Zoodles**

Preparation Time: 15 minutes

Servings: 4

Ingredients:

- ✓ ¼ cup chopped sun-dried tomatoes
- ✓ 4 spiralized zucchini
- ✓ ½ cup pesto
- ✓ 2 avocados, sliced

Directions:

- ❖ Heat 1 tbsp olive oil in a skillet over medium heat. Add zoodles and cook for 4 minutes.

Ingredients:

- ✓ 1 cup kalamata olives, chopped
- ✓ ¼ cup chopped basil
- ✓ 2 tbsp olive oil

- ❖ Transfer to a plate. Stir in 1 tbsp of olive oil, the pesto, basil, tomatoes and olives. Add the avocado slices. Serve.

Nutrition: Calories 449; Net carbs 8.4g; Fat 42g; Protein 6g

VEGAN & VEGETARIAN RECIPES

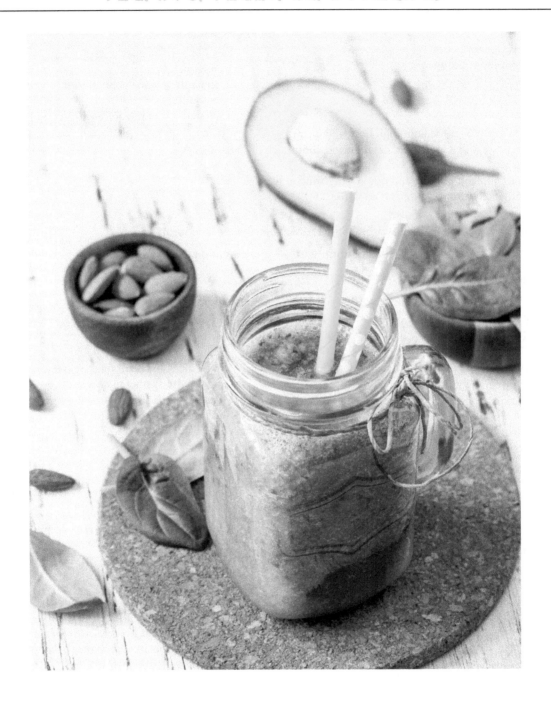

50) Briam with tomato sauce

Preparation Time: 40 minutes

Servings: 4

Ingredients:

- ✓ 3 tbsp olive oil
- ✓ 1 large eggplant, halved and sliced
- ✓ 1 large onion, thinly sliced
- ✓ 3 garlic cloves, sliced
- ✓ 2 tomatoes, diced
- ✓ 1 rutabaga, diced

Directions:

- ❖ Preheat oven to 400°F. Heat the olive oil in a skillet over medium heat and fry the eggplant and zucchini slices for 6 minutes until golden brown. Remove them to a casserole dish and arrange them in a single layer.

Ingredients:

- ✓ 1 cup unsweetened tomato sauce
- ✓ 4 zucchini, sliced
- ✓ ¼ cup water
- ✓ Salt and black pepper to taste
- ✓ ¼ tsp dried oregano
- ✓ 2 tbsp fresh parsley, chopped
- ❖ Sauté the onion and garlic in the oil for 3 minutes. Remove to a bowl. Add the tomatoes, rutabaga, tomato sauce and water and mix well. Stir in salt, pepper, oregano and parsley. Pour the mixture over the eggplant and zucchini. Place the dish in the oven and bake for 25-30 minutes. Serve the briam hot.

Nutrition: Calories Calories 365, Fat 12g, Net Carbohydrates 12.5g, Protein 11.3g

51) Creamy vegetable stew

Preparation Time: 25 minutes

Servings: 4

Ingredients:

- ✓ 2 tbsp ghee
- ✓ 1 tbsp onion and garlic puree
- ✓ 2 medium carrots, shredded
- ✓ 1 head of cauliflower, cut into florets

Directions:

- ❖ Melt ghee in a saucepan over medium heat and sauté onion and garlic puree to be fragrant, 2 minutes. Stir in carrots, cauliflower and green beans for 5 minutes. Season with salt and black pepper.

Ingredients:

- ✓ 2 cups green beans, cut in half
- ✓ Salt and black pepper to taste
- ✓ 1 cup water
- ✓ 1 ½ cups heavy cream
- ❖ Pour in water, stir again and cook over low heat for 15 minutes. Stir in the heavy cream to incorporate and turn off the heat. Serve the stew with almond flour bread.

Nutrition: Calories 310, fat 26.4g, net carbs 6g, protein 8g

52) Tempeh kabobs with vegetables

Preparation Time: 30 minutes + cooling time

Servings: 4

Ingredients:

- ✓ 2 tbsp ghee
- ✓ 1 tbsp onion and garlic puree
- ✓ 2 medium carrots, shredded
- ✓ 1 head of cauliflower, cut into florets

Directions:

- ❖ Melt ghee in a saucepan over medium heat and sauté onion and garlic puree to be fragrant, 2 minutes. Stir in carrots, cauliflower and green beans for 5 minutes. Season with salt and black pepper.

Ingredients:

- ✓ 2 cups green beans, cut in half
- ✓ Salt and black pepper to taste
- ✓ 1 cup water
- ✓ 1 ½ cups heavy cream
- ❖ Pour in water, stir again and cook over low heat for 15 minutes. Stir in the heavy cream to incorporate and turn off the heat. Serve the stew with almond flour bread.

Nutrition: Calories Calories 228, Fat 15g, Net Carbohydrates 3.6g, Protein 13.2g

53) Tempeh kabobs with vegetables

Preparation Time: 30 minutes + cooling time

Servings: 4

Ingredients:
- ✓ 1 yellow bell pepper, cut into pieces
- ✓ 10 ounces tempeh, cut into pieces
- ✓ 1 red onion, cut into pieces

Directions:
- ❖ Bring the 1 ½ cups of water to a boil in a pot over medium heat, and once it's cooked, turn off the heat and add the tempeh. Cover the pot and allow the tempeh to steam for 5 minutes to remove the bitterness. Drain. Pour barbecue sauce into a bowl, add tempeh and coat with sauce. Refrigerate for 2 hours.

Ingredients:
- ✓ 1 red bell bell pepper, cut into pieces
- ✓ 2 tbsp olive oil
- ✓ 1 cup unsweetened barbecue sauce
- ❖ Preheat grill to 350°F. Thread the tempeh, yellow bell pepper, red bell pepper and onion onto skewers. Brush the grill grate with olive oil, place the skewers on and brush with the barbecue sauce. Cook skewers for 3 minutes on each side, rotating and brushing with more barbecue sauce. Serve.

Nutrition: Calories Calories 228, Fat 15g, Net Carbohydrates 3.6g, Protein 13.2g

54) Cauliflower and Gouda Cheese Casserole

Preparation Time: 25 minutes

Servings: 4

Ingredients:
- ✓ 2 heads of cauliflower, cut into florets
- ✓ 2 tbsp olive oil
- ✓ 2 tbsp melted butter
- ✓ 1 white onion, chopped

Directions:
- ❖ Preheat oven to 350°F. Place cauli florets in a large microwave-safe bowl. Sprinkle with a little water and steam in the microwave for 4 to 5 minutes. Heat the olive oil in a saucepan over medium heat and sauté the onion for 3 minutes. Add the cauliflower, season with salt and pepper and stir in the almond milk.

Ingredients:
- ✓ Salt and black pepper to taste
- ✓ ¼ cup almond milk
- ✓ ½ cup almond flour
- ✓ 1 ½ cups gouda cheese, grated
- ❖ Cook over low heat for 3 minutes. Mix the melted butter with the almond flour. Stir in the cauliflower and half of the cheese. Sprinkle the top with the remaining cheese and bake for 10 minutes until the cheese is melted and golden brown on top. Plate the oven and serve with the salad.

Nutrition: Calories 215, Fat 15g, Net Carbs 4g, Protein 12g

55) Roasted Asparagus with Spicy Eggplant Sauce

Preparation Time: 35 minutes   **Servings: 6**

Ingredients:
- 1 ½ pounds asparagus, chopped
- ¼ cup + 2 tbsp olive oil
- ½ tsp paprika
- Eggplant Sauce
- 1 pound of eggplant
- ½ cup shallots, chopped

Directions:
- Preheat oven to 390°F. Line a parchment paper on a baking sheet. Add the asparagus. Season with 2 tbsp olive oil, paprika, black pepper and salt. Roast until cooked through, 9 minutes. Remove.
- Place the eggplant on a cookie sheet lined baking sheet. Bake in the oven for about 20 minutes.

Ingredients:
- 2 cloves garlic, minced
- 1 tbsp fresh lemon juice
- ½ tsp chili pepper
- Salt and black pepper to taste
- ¼ cup fresh cilantro, chopped

- Allow eggplant to cool. Peel them and discard the stems. Heat the remaining olive oil in a skillet over medium heat and add the garlic and shallots. Sauté for 3 minutes until tender.
- In a food processor, put together the black pepper, roasted eggplant, salt, lemon juice, shallot mixture, and red pepper. Add the cilantro and serve alongside the roasted asparagus spears.

Nutrition: Calories 149; Fat: 12.1g, Net Carbohydrates: 9g, Protein: 3.6g

56) Cook the squash

Preparation Time: 45 minutes   **Servings: 6**

Ingredients:
- 3 large pumpkins, peeled and sliced
- 1 cup almond flour
- 1 cup grated mozzarella cheese

Directions:
- Preheat oven to 350°F. Arrange the squash slices in a baking dish and drizzle with olive oil.

Ingredients:
- 3 tbsp olive oil
- ½ cup fresh parsley, chopped

- Bake for 35 minutes. Mix almond flour, mozzarella cheese and parsley and pour over squash. Return to oven and bake for another 5 minutes until top is golden brown. Serve warm.

Nutrition: Calories 125, Fat 4.8g, Net Carbs 5.7g, Protein 2.7g

57) Cremini Mushroom Stroganoff

Preparation Time: 25 minutes   **Servings: 4**

Ingredients:
- 3 tbsp butter
- 1 white onion, chopped
- 4 cups cremini mushrooms, diced

Directions:
- Melt the butter in a saucepan over medium heat and sauté the onion for 3 minutes until soft. Add the mushrooms and cook until tender, about 5 minutes. Add 2 cups of water and bring to a boil.

Ingredients:
- ½ cup heavy cream
- ½ cup Parmesan cheese, grated
- 1 ½ tbsp dried mixed herbs
- Cook for 10-15 minutes until the water reduces slightly. Pour in the heavy cream and Parmesan cheese. Stir to dissolve the cheese. Add the dried herbs and season. Simmer for 5 minutes. Serve hot.

Nutrition: Calories 284, Fat 28g, Net Carbs 1.5g, Protein 8g

58) Portobello Mushroom Burger

Preparation Time: 15 minutes

Servings: 4

Ingredients:

- ✓ 8 large portobello mushroom caps
- ✓ 1 minced garlic clove
- ✓ ½ cup of mayonnaise
- ✓ ½ tsp salt
- ✓ 4 tbsp olive oil
- ✓ ½ cup roasted red peppers, sliced

Directions:

- ❖ Preheat a grill over medium-high heat. In a bowl, crush the garlic with the salt using the back of a spoon. Stir in half the oil and brush the mushrooms and halloumi cheese with the mixture.
- ❖ Place the "sandwiches" on the skillet and grill them on both sides for 8 minutes until tender.

Ingredients:

- ✓ 2 medium tomatoes, chopped
- ✓ 4 halloumi slices, half-inch thick
- ✓ 1 tbsp red wine vinegar
- ✓ 2 tbsp Kalamata olives, chopped
- ✓ ½ tsp dried oregano
- ✓ 2 cups spinach
- ❖ Add the halloumi cheese slices to the grill. Cook for 2 minutes per side or until golden brown marks appear on the grill.
- ❖ In a bowl, mix red peppers, tomatoes, olives, vinegar, oregano, spinach and remaining olive oil; toss to coat. Spread mayonnaise on 4 mushroom "sandwiches", top with a slice of halloumi, a scoop of greens and top with remaining mushrooms. Serve and enjoy!

Nutrition: Calories 339, Fat 29.4g, Net Carbs 3.5g, Protein 10g

59) Sriracha tofu with yogurt sauce

Preparation Time: 40 minutes

Servings: 4

Ingredients:

- ✓ 12 ounces tofu, pressed and sliced
- ✓ 1 cup green onions, chopped
- ✓ 1 clove garlic, minced
- ✓ 2 tbsp vinegar
- ✓ 1 tbsp sriracha sauce
- ✓ 2 tbsp olive oil

Directions:

- ❖ Place the tofu slices, garlic, sriracha sauce, vinegar and green onions in a bowl. Let stand for 30 minutes. Place a nonstick skillet over medium heat and add oil to heat. Cook the tofu for 5 minutes until golden brown.

Ingredients:

- ✓ Yogurt Sauce
- ✓ 2 cloves garlic, crushed
- ✓ 2 tbsp fresh lemon juice
- ✓ Salt and black pepper to taste
- ✓ 1 tsp fresh dill
- ✓ 1 cup Greek yogurt
- ✓ 1 cucumber, shredded
- ❖ To make the sauce: In a bowl, mix garlic, salt, yogurt, black pepper, lemon juice and dill. Add shredded cucumber while stirring to combine. Serve tofu with a spoonful of yogurt sauce.

Nutrition: Calories 351; Fat: 25.9g, Net Carbohydrates: 8.1g, Protein: 17.5g

60) Jalapeño and Vegetable Stew

Preparation Time: 40 minutes

Servings: 4

Ingredients:

- ✓ 2 tbsp butter
- ✓ 1 cup leeks, chopped
- ✓ 1 clove garlic, minced
- ✓ ½ cup celery stalks, chopped
- ✓ ½ cup carrots, chopped
- ✓ 1 green bell bell pepper, chopped
- ✓ 1 jalapeño bell pepper, chopped
- ✓ 1 zucchini, chopped

Ingredients:

- ✓ 1 cup mushrooms, sliced
- ✓ 1 ½ cups vegetable broth
- ✓ 2 tomatoes, chopped
- ✓ 2 tbsp fresh parsley, chopped
- ✓ 2 bay leaves
- ✓ Salt and black pepper to taste
- ✓ 1 tbsp vinegar

Directions:

- ❖ Melt the butter in a saucepan over medium heat. Add the garlic and leeks and sauté for 3 minutes until soft and translucent. Add the celery, mushrooms, zucchini and carrots and sauté for another 5 minutes.

- ❖ Stir in the rest of the ingredients. Season with salt and pepper. Bring to a boil and simmer for 15-20 minutes or until cooked through. Divide among individual bowls and serve hot.

Nutrition: Calories 65; Fat: 2.7g, Net Carbohydrates: 9g, Protein: 2.7g

61) Raspberry and turmeric panna cotta

Preparation Time: 10 minutes + cooling time

Servings: 6

Ingredients:

- ✓ ½ tbsp unflavored vegetable gelatin powder
- ✓ 2 cups of coconut cream
- ✓ ¼ tsp vanilla extract
- ✓ 1 tsp turmeric

Ingredients:

- ✓ 1 tbsp erythritol
- ✓ 1 tbsp chopped toasted pecans
- ✓ 12 fresh raspberries

Directions:

- ❖ Mix the gelatin and ½ tbsp water and let it dissolve. Pour the coconut cream, vanilla extract, turmeric and erythritol into a saucepan and bring to a boil; simmer for 2 minutes. Turn off the heat. Stir in gelatin.

- ❖ Pour into 6 glasses, cover with plastic wrap and refrigerate for 2 hours. Top with pecans and raspberries and serve.

Nutrition: Calories 270; Net Carbs 3g; Fat 27g; Protein 4g

62) Mixed Berry Yogurt Ice Pops

Preparation Time: 2 minutes + cooling time

Servings: 6

Ingredients:

- ✓ 2/3 cup frozen strawberries and blueberries, thawed
- ✓ 2/3 cup avocado, halved, pitted
- ✓ 1 cup plain yogurt

Ingredients:

- ✓ ½ cup cream of coconut
- ✓ 1 tsp vanilla extract

Directions:

- ❖ Pour avocado, berries, yogurt, coconut cream and vanilla extract into a blender.

- ❖ Process until smooth. Pour into ice pop sleeves and freeze for 8 hours. Serve when ready to serve.

Nutrition: Calories 80; Net carbs 4g; Fat 5g; Protein 2g

SNACK & SIDE DISHES

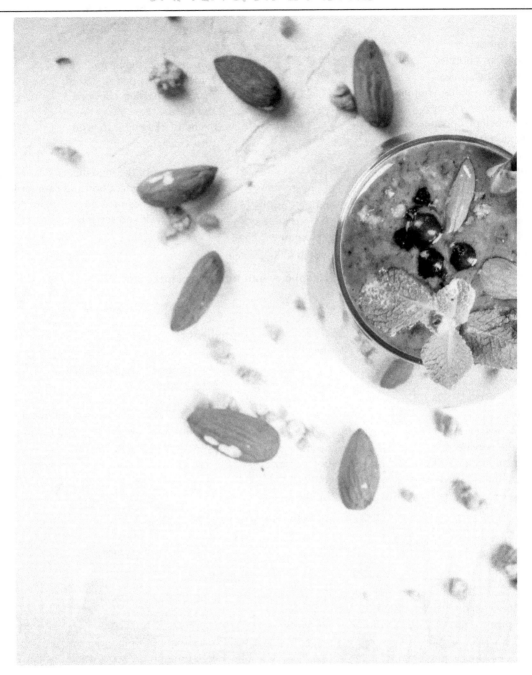

63) Chicken with Cheese

Preparation Time: 20 minutes

Servings: 4

Ingredients:

✓ ¼ tsp garlic powder
✓ 4 ounces fontina cheese

Directions:

❖ Pound chicken until 1/2 inch thick. Season with garlic powder. Cut fontina cheese into 8 strips.

Ingredients:

✓ 4 tenders raw chicken
✓ 4 slices raw ham

❖ Place one slice of ham on a flat surface. Place tender chicken on top. Top with a strip of fontina cheese. Roll up chicken and secure with skewers. Grill the strips for 3 minutes per side. Serve.

Nutrition: Calories 174; Net carbs: 1g; Fat: 10g; Protein: 17g

64) Brussels sprouts and bacon rolls

Preparation Time: 15 minutes

Servings: 4

Ingredients:

✓ 16 Brussels sprouts, cut
✓ 8 slices of bacon

Directions:

❖ Preheat oven to 420 F. Line a baking sheet with baking paper. Cut the bacon slices in half. Wrap each Brussels sprout with a strip of bacon.

Ingredients:

✓ 1/8 tsp chili pepper

❖ Transfer the wraps to the baking sheet and bake for 25-30 until crispy. Sprinkle with chili powder and serve immediately.

Nutrition: Calories 193; Net carbs 1.6g; Fat 14g; Protein 12g

65) Waffle sandwiches with gruyere and ham

Preparation Time: 20 minutes

Servings: 4

Ingredients:

✓ 4 slices smoked ham, chopped
✓ 4 tbsp butter, softened
✓ ½ cup Gruyere cheese, grated
✓ 6 eggs

Directions:

❖ In a bowl, mix the eggs, baking powder, thyme and butter. Place a waffle iron over medium heat, add ¼ cup of the batter and cook for 6 minutes until golden brown. Do the same with the remaining batter until you have 8 thin waffles.

Ingredients:

✓ ½ tsp baking powder
✓ ½ tsp dried thyme
✓ 4 slices tomato

❖ Lay a slice of tomato on one waffle, followed by a slice of ham, then top with ¼ of the grated cheese. Cover with another waffle, place the sandwich in the waffle iron and cook until the cheese melts. Repeat with remaining ingredients.

Nutrition: Calories 276; Net carbs 3.1g; Fat 22g; Protein 16g

66) Baked chorizo with ricotta cheese

Preparation Time: 30 minutes   **Servings: 6**

Ingredients:
- ✓ 7 ounces Spanish chorizo, sliced
- ✓ 4 ounces ricotta cheese, crumbled

Directions:
- ❖ Preheat oven to 325 F. Spread chorizo on a wax paper-lined baking sheet and bake for 15 minutes until crispy

Ingredients:
- ✓ ¼ cup chopped parsley

- ❖ Remove from oven and allow to cool. Arrange on a serving platter. Add ricotta cheese and parsley.

Nutrition: Calories 172; Net carbohydrates: 0.2g; Fat: 13g; Protein: 5g

67) Mediterranean Salad

Preparation Time: 10 minutes   **Servings: 4**

Ingredients:
- ✓ 3 tomatoes, sliced
- ✓ 1 large avocado, sliced
- ✓ 8 kalamata olives

Directions:
- ❖ Arrange the tomato slices on a serving platter and place the avocado slices in the center.

Ingredients:
- ✓ ¼ lb buffalo mozzarella, sliced
- ✓ 2 tbsp pesto sauce
- ✓ 1 tbsp olive oil
- ❖ Arrange the olives around the avocado slices and drop mozzarella pieces onto the serving plate. Drizzle the pesto sauce and olive oil over everything and serve.

Nutrition: Calories 290, Fat: 25g, Net carbs: 4.3g, Protein: 9g

68) Tuna salad with lettuce and olives

Preparation Time: 5 minutes   **Servings: 2**

Ingredients:
- ✓ 1 cup canned tuna, drained
- ✓ 1 tsp of onion flakes
- ✓ 3 tbsp mayonnaise

Directions:
- ❖ Combine tuna, mayonnaise and lime juice in a small bowl. Stir to combine. In a salad bowl, arrange shredded lettuce and onion flakes.

Ingredients:
- ✓ 1 cup romaine lettuce, shredded
- ✓ 1 tbsp lime juice
- ✓ 6 black olives, pitted and sliced
- ❖ Spread the tuna mixture over the top. Top with black olives and serve.

Nutrition: Calories 248, Fat: 20g, Net Carbs: 2g, Protein: 18.5g

69) Cobb egg salad in lettuce cups

Preparation Time: 25 minutes

Servings: 4

Ingredients:

- ✓ 1 head of green lettuce, firm leaves removed for cups
- ✓ 2 chicken breasts, cut into pieces
- ✓ 1 tbsp olive oil
- ✓ Salt and black pepper to taste

Directions:

- ❖ Preheat oven to 400°F. Place chicken in a bowl, drizzle with olive oil and sprinkle with salt and black pepper. Cough to coat. Place the chicken on a baking sheet and spread it out evenly. Slide the baking sheet into the oven and bake the chicken until cooked through and golden brown for 8 minutes, stirring once.

Ingredients:

- ✓ 6 large eggs
- ✓ 2 tomatoes, seeded, chopped
- ✓ 6 tbsp Greek yogurt

- ❖ Boil the eggs in salted water for 10 minutes. Allow them to cool, peel and cut into pieces. Transfer to a salad bowl. Remove the chicken from the oven and add it to the salad bowl. Include the tomatoes and Greek yogurt and toss to combine. Layer 2 lettuce leaves each as cups and fill with 2 tbsp of egg salad each. Serve.

Nutrition: Calories 325, Fat 24.5g, Net Carbs 4g, Protein 21g

70) Blue Cheese Chicken Salad

Preparation Time: 15 minutes

Servings: 4

Ingredients:

- ✓ 1 chicken breast, flattened
- ✓ Salt and black pepper to taste
- ✓ 4 tbsp olive oil

Directions:

- ❖ Season the chicken with salt and black pepper. Heat half of the olive oil in a skillet over medium heat and fry the chicken for 4 minutes on both sides until golden brown. Remove and let cool before slicing.

Ingredients:

- ✓ 1 pound spinach and spring mix
- ✓ 1 tbsp red wine vinegar
- ✓ 1 cup blue cheese, crumbled
- ❖ In a salad bowl, combine the spinach and spring mix with the remaining olive oil, red wine vinegar and salt and mix well. Top the salad with the chicken slices and sprinkle with blue cheese. Serve.

Nutrition: Calories 286, Fat 23g, Net Carbs 4g, Protein 14g

71) Arugula Shrimp Salad with Mayo Dressing

Preparation Time: 15 minutes

Servings: 4

Ingredients:

- ✓ 4 cups arugula
- ✓ ½ cup mayonnaise
- ✓ 3 tbsp olive oil
- ✓ 1 pound shrimp, peeled and deveined
- ✓ 1 tsp Dijon mustard

Directions:

- ❖ Mix the mayonnaise, lemon juice, garlic powder and mustard in a small bowl until smooth and creamy. Set aside until ready to use. Heat 2 tbsp olive oil in a skillet over medium heat. Add shrimp, season with salt and pepper, and fry for 3 minutes on each side until shrimp are pink. Set aside on a plate.

Ingredients:

- ✓ Salt to taste
- ✓ ½ tsp chili pepper
- ✓ 2 tbsp lemon juice
- ✓ ½ tsp garlic powder

- ❖ Place arugula in a serving bowl and pour mayo dressing over salad. Toss with 2 tbsp until mixed. Divide salad among 4 plates and top with shrimp. Serve immediately.

Nutrition: Calories 215, Fat 20.3g, Net Carbs 2g, Protein 8g

72) Lobster salad with pink sauce

Preparation Time: 10 minutes

Servings: 4

Ingredients:
- ✓ 2 hard-boiled eggs, sliced
- ✓ 1 cucumber, peeled and chopped
- ✓ ½ cup black olives
- ✓ 2 cups cooked lobster meat, diced
- ✓ 1 head of iceberg lettuce, shredded

Ingredients:
- ✓ ½ cup mayonnaise
- ✓ ¼ tsp celery seed
- ✓ Salt to taste
- ✓ 2 tbsp lemon juice
- ✓ ½ tbsp unsweetened ketchup
- ✓ ¼ tsp dark rum

Directions:
- ❖ Combine the lettuce, cucumber, and lobster meat in a large bowl. Whisk together the mayonnaise, celery seed, ketchup, rum, salt and lemon juice in another bowl.

- ❖ Pour dressing over salad and toss gently to combine. Top with olives and sliced eggs and serve.

Nutrition: Calories 256, Fat: 15g, Net Carbs: 4.3g, Protein: 17.9g

73) Traditional Greek Salad

Preparation Time: 10 minutes

Servings: 4

Ingredients:
- ✓ 5 tomatoes, chopped
- ✓ 1 large cucumber, chopped
- ✓ 1 green bell pepper, chopped
- ✓ 1 small red onion, chopped
- ✓ 10 Kalamata olives, chopped

Ingredients:
- ✓ 4 tbsp capers
- ✓ 1 cup feta cheese, cubed
- ✓ 2 tbsp olive oil
- ✓ Salt to taste

Directions:
- ❖ Place the tomatoes, bell bell pepper, cucumber, onion, feta cheese, salt, capers and olive oil olives in a bowl.

- ❖ Stir to combine well. Divide salad among plates, top with Kalamata olives and serve.

Nutrition: Calories 323, Fat: 28g, Net Carbs: 8g, Protein: 9.3g

74) Mozzarella and tomato salad with anchovies and olives

Preparation Time: 10 minutes

Servings: 2

Ingredients:
- ✓ 1 large tomato, sliced
- ✓ 4 basil leaves
- ✓ 8 slices of mozzarella
- ✓ 2 tbsp olive oil

Ingredients:
- ✓ 2 canned anchovies, chopped
- ✓ 1 tsp balsamic vinegar
- ✓ 4 black olives, pitted and sliced
- ✓ Salt to taste
- ❖ Add the anchovies and olives on top. Drizzle with olive oil and vinegar. Sprinkle with salt and serve.

Directions:
- ❖ Arrange the tomato slices on a serving platter. Place the mozzarella slices on top and top with the basil.

Nutrition: Calories 430, Fat: 26.8g, Net Carbohydrates: 2.4g, Protein:38.8g

75) **Strawberry salad with cheese and almonds**

Preparation Time: 20 minutes

Servings: 2

Ingredients:
- ✓ 4 cups cabbage, chopped
- ✓ 4 strawberries, sliced
- ✓ ½ cup almonds, slivered

Directions:
- ❖ Preheat oven to 400°F. Arrange grated goat cheese in two circles on two pieces of parchment paper. Place in the oven and bake for 10 minutes. Find two equal bowls, place them upside down and carefully place the parchment paper on top to give the cheese a bowl-like shape.

Ingredients:
- ✓ 1 ½ cups hard goat cheese, grated
- ✓ 4 tbsp raspberry vinaigrette
- ✓ Salt and black pepper to taste
- ❖ Let cool like this for 15 minutes.
- ❖ Divide the cabbage between the bowls, sprinkle with salt and pepper, and drizzle with the vinaigrette. Stir to coat. Top with almonds and strawberries. Serve immediately.

Nutrition: Calories 445, Fat: 34.2g, Net Carbohydrates: 5.3g, Protein: 33g

76) **Spring salad with cheese balls**

Preparation Time: 20 minutes

Servings: 6

Ingredients:
- ✓ Cheese balls
- ✓ 3 eggs
- ✓ 1 cup feta cheese, crumbled
- ✓ ½ cup Pecorino cheese, crumbled
- ✓ 1 cup Almond Flour
- ✓ 1 tbsp flax meal
- ✓ Salt and black pepper to taste
- ✓ Salad
- ✓ 1 head Iceberg lettuce, leaves pulled apart
- ✓ ½ cup cucumber, thinly sliced

Directions:
- ❖ Preheat oven to 390°F. In a bowl, mix all the ingredients for the cheese balls. Form balls with the mixture. Place the balls on a lined baking sheet. Bake for 10 minutes until crispy.

Ingredients:
- ✓ 2 tomatoes, seeded and chopped
- ✓ ½ cup red onion, thinly sliced
- ✓ ½ cup radishes, thinly sliced
- ✓ ⅓ cup mayonnaise
- ✓ 1 tsp mustard
- ✓ 1 tsp paprika
- ✓ 1 tsp oregano
- ✓ Salt to taste

- ❖ Arrange lettuce leaves on a large salad plate. Add radishes, tomatoes, cucumbers and red onion. In a small bowl, mix mayonnaise, paprika, salt, oregano and mustard. Sprinkle the mixture over the vegetables. Add cheese balls on top and serve.

Nutrition: Calories: 234; Fat 16.7g, Net Carbohydrates 7.9g, Protein 12.4g

77) **Green mackerel salad**

Preparation Time: 25 minutes

Servings: 4

Ingredients:
- ✓ 4 oz smoked mackerel, flaked
- ✓ 2 eggs
- ✓ 1 tbsp coconut oil
- ✓ 1 cup green beans, chopped
- ✓ 1 avocado, sliced

Directions:
- ❖ In a bowl, whisk together the lemon juice, olive oil, salt and pepper. Set aside. Cook green beans in

Ingredients:
- ✓ 4 cups mixed salad
- ✓ 2 tbsp olive oil
- ✓ 1 tbsp lemon juice
- ✓ Salt and black pepper to taste

- ❖ Add the eggs to the pot and cook for 8-10 minutes. Transfer the eggs to an ice water bath, peel the shells and slice. Place the mixed green salad in a serving bowl and add the green beans and smoked

boiling salted water over medium heat for about 3 minutes. Remove with a slotted spoon and let cool.

mackerel. Pour in the dressing and toss to coat. Top with sliced egg and avocado and serve.

Nutrition: Calories 356, Fat: 31.9g, Net Carbs: 0.8g, Protein: 1.3g

78) **Grilled Steak Salad with Pickled Peppers**

Preparation Time: 15 minutes

Servings: 4

Ingredients:
- ½ lb skirt steak, sliced
- Salt and black pepper to taste
- 3 tbsp olive oil
- 1 head romaine lettuce, torn

Directions:
- Brush the steak slices with olive oil and season them with salt and black pepper on both sides. Heat a grill pan over high heat and cook the steaks on each side for about 5-6 minutes. Remove to a bowl.

Ingredients:
- 3 pickled peppers, chopped
- 2 tbsp red wine vinegar
- ½ cup queso fresco, crumbled
- 1 tbsp green olives, pitted, sliced
- ❖ Mix the lettuce, pickled peppers, remaining olive oil and vinegar in a salad bowl. Add beef and sprinkle with queso fresco and green olives. Serve.

Nutrition: Calories 315, Fat 26g, Net Carbs 2g, Protein 18g

79) **Cauliflower salad with shrimp and avocado**

Preparation Time: 30 minutes

Servings: 6

Ingredients:
- 1 head cauliflower, florets only
- 1 pound medium shrimp, shelled
- ¼ cup + 1 tbsp olive oil
- 1 avocado, chopped

Directions:
- Heat 1 tbsp olive oil in a skillet and cook the shrimp for 8 minutes. Microwave the cauliflower for 5 minutes

Ingredients:
- 2 tbsp fresh dill, chopped
- ¼ cup lemon juice
- 2 tbsp lemon zest
- Salt and black pepper to taste
- ❖ Place the shrimp, cauliflower, and avocado in a bowl. Whisk the remaining olive oil, lemon zest, juice, dill, salt and pepper in another bowl. Pour over the dressing, toss to combine and serve immediately.

Nutrition: Calories 214, Fat: 17g, Net Carbs: 5g, Protein: 15g

80) **Caesar Salad with Smoked Salmon and Poached Eggs**

Preparation Time: 15 minutes

Servings: 4

Ingredients:
- 8 eggs
- 2 cups torn romaine lettuce
- ½ cup smoked salmon, chopped

Directions:
- Bring a pot of water to a boil and pour in the vinegar. Crack each egg into a small bowl and gently slide it into the water. Soak for 2 to 3 minutes, remove with a slotted spoon and transfer to a paper towel to remove excess water and plate. Poach the remaining 7 eggs.

Ingredients:
- 6 slices of bacon
- 2 tbsp low-carb Caesar dressing
- 1 tbsp white wine vinegar
- ❖ Place the bacon in a skillet and fry it over medium heat until browned and crispy, about 6 minutes, turning once. Remove, let cool and cut into small pieces. Mix the lettuce, smoked salmon, bacon and Caesar dressing in a salad bowl. Top with two eggs each and serve immediately or chilled.

Nutrition: Calories 260, Fat 21g, Net Carbs 5g, Protein 8g

81) Bacon and Spinach Salad

Preparation Time: 20 minutes

Servings: 4

Ingredients:

✓ 1 avocado, chopped
✓ 1 avocado, sliced
✓ 1 spring onion, sliced
✓ 4 slices bacon, chopped
✓ 2 cups spinach
✓ 2 small heads of lettuce, chopped

Directions:

❖ Place a skillet over medium heat and cook the bacon for 5 minutes until crispy. Remove to a paper towel-lined plate to drain. Boil the eggs in boiling salted water for 10 minutes. Let them cool, peel and chop them.

Ingredients:

✓ 2 eggs
✓ 3 tbsp olive oil
✓ 1 tbsp Dijon mustard
✓ 1 tbsp apple cider vinegar
✓ Salt to taste

❖ Combine the spinach, lettuce, eggs, chopped avocado and spring onion in a large bowl. Whisk together the olive oil, mustard, apple cider vinegar and salt in another bowl. Pour the dressing over the salad and toss to combine. Top with the sliced avocado and bacon and serve.

Nutrition: Calories 350, Fat: 33g, Net Carbs: 3.4g, Protein: 7g

82) Brussels Sprouts Salad with Pecorino Cheese

Preparation Time: 35 minutes

Servings: 6

Ingredients:

✓ 2 lb Brussels sprouts, halved
✓ 3 tbsp olive oil
✓ Salt and black pepper to taste

Directions:

❖ Preheat the oven to 400°F. Toss brussels sprouts with olive oil, salt, black pepper and balsamic vinegar in a bowl. Spread on a baking sheet in an even layer.

Ingredients:

✓ 2 tbsp balsamic vinegar
✓ ¼ head red cabbage, shredded
✓ 1 cup Pecorino cheese, shredded
❖ Bake until tender on the inside and crisp on the outside, about 20-25 minutes. Transfer to a salad bowl and add the red cabbage. Stir until well combined. Sprinkle with cheese, divide salad on serving plates and serve.

Nutrition: Calories 210, Fat 18g, Net Carbs 6g, Protein 4g

83) Pork Burger Salad with Yellow Cheddar

Preparation Time: 25 minutes

Servings: 4

Ingredients:

✓ ½ pound ground pork
✓ Salt and black pepper to taste
✓ 2 tbsp olive oil
✓ 2 hearts of romaine lettuce, torn

Directions:

❖ Season the pork with salt and black pepper, mix it, and make medium-sized patties. Heat the butter in a skillet over medium heat and fry the patties on both sides for 10 minutes until golden brown and cooked through on the inside.

Ingredients:

✓ 2 firm tomatoes, sliced
✓ ¼ red onion, sliced
✓ 3 ounces yellow cheddar cheese, grated
✓ 2 tbsp butter
❖ Transfer to a rack to drain off the oil. Once cooled, cut into quarters.
❖ Mix the lettuce, tomatoes, and red onion in a salad bowl, drizzle with olive oil and salt. Stir and add the pork on top. Top with cheese and serve.

Nutrition: Calories 310, Fat 23g, Net Carbs 2g, Protein 22g

84) **Italian style green salad**

Preparation Time: 15 minutes

Servings: 4

Ingredients:
- ✓ 2 (8 oz) package mixed salad
- ✓ 8 strips of bacon
- ✓ 1 cup gorgonzola cheese, crumbled

Directions:
- ❖ Fry the bacon strips in a skillet over medium heat for 6 minutes, until golden brown and crispy. Remove to a paper towel-lined plate to drain. Chop when cooled. Pour the green salad into a serving bowl.

Ingredients:
- ✓ 1 tbsp white wine vinegar
- ✓ 3 tbsp extra virgin olive oil
- ✓ Salt and black pepper to taste
- ❖ In a small bowl, whisk the white wine vinegar, olive oil, salt and pepper. Drizzle the dressing over the salad and toss to coat. Top with gorgonzola cheese and bacon. Divide salad among plates and serve.

Nutrition: Calories 205, Fat 20g, Net Carbs 2g, Protein 4g

85) **Broccoli Salad Salad with Mustard Vinaigrette**

Preparation Time: 10 minutes

Servings: 6

Ingredients:
- ✓ ½ tsp granulated sugar swerve
- ✓ 1 tbsp Dijon mustard
- ✓ 2 tbsp olive oil
- ✓ 4 cups broccoli salad
- ✓ ⅓ cup mayonnaise

Directions:
- ❖ In a bowl, place the mayonnaise, Dijon mustard, sugar swerve, olive oil, celery seeds, vinegar and salt and whisk until well combined.

Ingredients:
- ✓ 1 tsp celery seeds
- ✓ 2 tbsp slivered almonds
- ✓ 1 ½ tbsp apple cider vinegar
- ✓ Salt to taste

- ❖ Place the broccoli salad in a large salad bowl. Pour the vinaigrette over the top. Stir to coat. Sprinkle with slivered almonds and serve immediately.

Nutrition: Calories 110, Fat: 10g, Net Carbs: 2g, Protein: 3g

86) **Warm Artichoke Salad**

Preparation Time: 30 minutes

Servings: 4

Ingredients:
- ✓ 6 baby artichokes
- ✓ 6 cups water
- ✓ 1 tbsp lemon juice
- ✓ ¼ cup cherry peppers, halved
- ✓ ¼ cup pitted olives, sliced
- ✓ ¼ cup olive oil

Directions:
- ❖ Combine the water and salt in a saucepan over medium heat. Trim and halve the artichokes. Add them to the pot and bring to a boil. Lower the heat and simmer for 20 minutes until tender.

Ingredients:
- ✓ ¼ tsp lemon zest
- ✓ 2 tbsp balsamic vinegar, unsweetened
- ✓ 1 tbsp chopped dill
- ✓ Salt and black pepper to taste
- ✓ 1 tbsp capers
- ✓ ¼ tsp caper brine
- ❖ Combine the rest of the ingredients, except the olives, in a bowl. Drain and arrange the artichokes on a serving platter. Pour prepared mixture over them; toss to combine well. Serve topped with the olives.

Nutrition: Calories 170, Fat: 13g, Net carbs: 5g, Protein: 1g

87) Squid salad with cucumbers and chili sauce

Preparation Time: 30 minutes   **Servings: 4**

Ingredients:

- ✓ 4 tubes of squid, cut into strips
- ✓ ½ cup mint leaves
- ✓ 2 cucumbers, halved, cut into strips
- ✓ ½ cup cilantro, stalks reserved
- ✓ ½ red onion, finely sliced
- ✓ Salt and black pepper to taste

Ingredients:

- ✓ 1 tsp fish sauce
- ✓ 1 red chili pepper, coarsely chopped
- ✓ 1 garlic clove
- ✓ 2 limes, squeezed
- ✓ 1 tbsp fresh parsley, chopped
- ✓ 1 tsp olive oil

Directions:

- ❖ In a salad bowl, mix mint leaves, cucumber strips, cilantro leaves and red onion. Season with salt, black pepper and a little olive oil; set aside. In a mortar, pound the cilantro stalks and red pepper to form a paste using the pestle. Add the fish sauce and lime juice and stir with the pestle.

- ❖ Heat a frying pan over medium heat. Brown the squid on both sides until lightly browned, about 5 minutes. Pour the calamari over the salad and drizzle with the chili dressing. Stir to coat, garnish with parsley and serve.

Nutrition: Calories 318, Fat 22.5g, Net Carbohydrates 2.1g, Protein 24.6g

88) Spinach and Turnip Salad with Bacon

Preparation Time: 40 minutes   **Servings: 4**

Ingredients:

- ✓ 2 turnips, cut into wedges
- ✓ 1 tsp olive oil
- ✓ 1 cup baby spinach, chopped
- ✓ 3 radishes, sliced
- ✓ 3 slices turkey bacon
- ✓ 4 tbsp sour cream

Ingredients:

- ✓ 2 tbsp mustard seed
- ✓ 1 tsp Dijon mustard
- ✓ 1 tbsp red wine vinegar
- ✓ Salt and black pepper to taste
- ✓ 1 tbsp chopped chives

Directions:

- ❖ Preheat oven to 400°F. Line a baking sheet with parchment paper, toss the turnips with salt and black pepper, drizzle with olive oil and bake for 25 minutes, turning halfway through. Allow to cool.

- ❖ Spread the spinach in the bottom of a salad bowl and top with the radishes. Remove the turnips to the salad bowl. Fry the bacon in a skillet over medium heat until crispy, about 5 minutes.
- ❖ Mix sour cream, mustard seeds, mustard, vinegar and salt with the bacon. Add a little water to deglaze the bottom of the pan. Pour the bacon mixture over the vegetables and scatter the chives. Serve.

Nutrition: Calories 193, Fat 18.3g, Net Carbohydrates 3.1g, Protein 9.5g

89) **Chicken Salad with Grapefruit and Cashews**

Preparation Time: 30 minutes + marinating time

Servings: 4

Ingredients:

- ✓ 1 grapefruit, peeled and segmented
- ✓ 1 chicken breast
- ✓ 4 green onions, sliced
- ✓ 10 ounces baby spinach
- ✓ 2 tbsp cashews

Directions:

- ❖ Toast cashews in a dry skillet over high heat for 2 minutes, shaking often. Set aside to cool, then cut them into small pieces. Preheat the grill to medium heat. Season the chicken with salt and pepper and brush it with a little olive oil.

Ingredients:

- ✓ 1 red chili pepper, thinly sliced
- ✓ 1 lemon, squeezed
- ✓ 3 tbsp olive oil
- ✓ Salt and black pepper to taste

- ❖ Grill for 4 minutes per side. Remove to a plate and let it rest for a few minutes before slicing.
- ❖ Arrange the spinach and green onions on a serving platter. Season with salt, remaining olive oil and lemon juice. Stir to coat. Top with the chicken, chili and chicken. Sprinkle with cashews and serve.

Nutrition: Calories 178, Fat: 13.5g, Net carbohydrates: 3.2g, Protein: 9.1g

90) **Cobb Salad with Blue Cheese Dressing**

Preparation Time: 30 minutes

Servings: 6

Ingredients:

- ✓ Dressing
- ✓ ½ cup buttermilk
- ✓ 1 cup mayonnaise
- ✓ 2 tbsp Worcestershire sauce
- ✓ ½ cup sour cream
- ✓ 1 cup blue cheese, crumbled
- ✓ 2 tbsp chives, chopped
- ✓ Salad
- ✓ 6 eggs
- ✓ 2 chicken breasts

Directions:

- ❖ In a bowl, whisk buttermilk, mayonnaise, Worcestershire sauce and sour cream. Stir in the blue cheese and chives. Refrigerate to chill until ready to use. Bring eggs to boil in salted water over medium heat for 10 minutes. Transfer to an ice bath to cool. Peel and chop. Set aside.
- ❖ Preheat a grill pan over high heat. Season chicken with salt and pepper. Grill for 3 minutes on each side. Remove to a plate to cool for 3 minutes and cut into pieces.

Ingredients:

- ✓ 5 strips of bacon
- ✓ 1 iceberg lettuce, chopped
- ✓ Salt and black pepper to taste
- ✓ 1 romaine lettuce, cut into pieces
- ✓ 1 bibb lettuce, core, leaves removed
- ✓ 2 avocados, pitted and diced
- ✓ 2 large tomatoes, chopped
- ✓ ½ cup blue cheese, crumbled
- ✓ 2 shallots, chopped

- ❖ . Fry the bacon in the same skillet until crispy, about 6 minutes. Remove, let cool for 2 minutes and cut into pieces.
- ❖ Arrange the lettuce leaves in a salad bowl and, in individual piles, add the avocado, tomatoes, eggs, bacon and chicken. Sprinkle the salad with the blue cheese, scallions and black pepper. Drizzle the blue cheese dressing over the salad and serve with low carb bread.

Nutrition: Calories 122, Fat 14g, Net Carbs 2g, Protein 23g

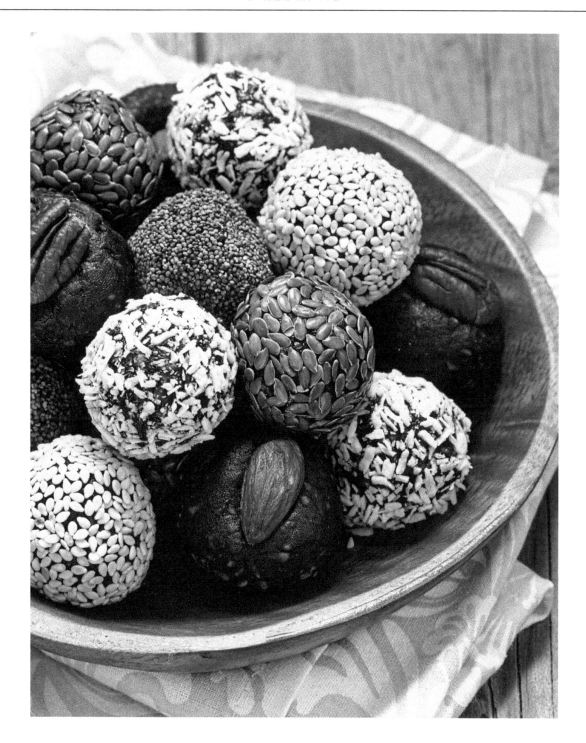

91) Merry Berry

Preparation Time: 6 minutes

Servings: 4

Ingredients:
- ✓ 1 cup strawberries + extra for garnish
- ✓ 1 ½ cups blackberries
- ✓ 1 cup blueberries

Directions:
- ❖ For extra strawberries for garnish, make a single deep cut on their sides; set aside. Add blackberries, strawberries, blueberries, beets and ice cubes to smoothie maker.

Ingredients:
- ✓ 2 small beets, peeled and chopped
- ✓ 2/3 cup ice cubes
- ✓ 1 lime, squeezed
- ❖ Blend ingredients on high speed until smooth and frothy, about 60 seconds. Add the lime juice and blend for 30 seconds more. Pour the drink into tall smoothie glasses, secure the reserved strawberries on the rim of each glass, stick a straw in and serve the drink immediately.

Nutrition: Calories 83, Fat 3g, Net Carbs 8g, Protein 2.7g

92) Cinnamon Cookies

Preparation Time: 25 minutes

Servings: 4

Ingredients:
- ✓ Cookies
- ✓ 2 cups almond flour
- ✓ ½ tsp baking soda
- ✓ ¾ cup sweetener
- ✓ ½ cup butter, softened

Directions:
- ❖ Preheat oven to 350°F. Combine all cookie ingredients in a bowl. Make 16 balls with the dough and flatten them with your hands. Combine the cinnamon and erythritol.

Ingredients:
- ✓ A pinch of salt
- ✓ Coating
- ✓ 2 tbsp erythritol sweetener
- ✓ 1 tsp cinnamon
- ❖ Dip the cookies into the cinnamon mixture and place them on a lined baking sheet. Bake for 15 minutes, until crispy.

Nutrition: Calories 134, Fat: 13g, Net Carbs: 1.5g, Protein: 3g

93) Vanilla Frappuccino

Preparation Time: 6 minutes

Servings: 4

Ingredients:
- ✓ 3 cups unsweetened vanilla almond milk, chilled Unsweetened chocolate chips for garnish
- ✓ 2 tbsp sugar swerve
- ✓ 1 ½ cups heavy cream, chilled

Directions:
- ❖ Combine almond milk, swerve sugar, heavy cream, vanilla bean and xanthan gum in blender and process on high speed for 1 minute until smooth.

Ingredients:
- ✓ 1 vanilla bean
- ✓ ¼ tsp xanthan gum
- ❖ Pour into tall shake glasses, sprinkle with chocolate chips and serve immediately.

Nutrition: Calories 193, Fat 14g, Net Carbs 6g, Protein 15g

94) **Peanut Butter Pecan Ice Cream**

Preparation Time: 36 minutes + cooling time

Servings: 4

Ingredients:

- ✓ ½ cup swerve confectioners sweetener
- ✓ 2 cups heavy cream
- ✓ 1 tbsp of erythritol
- ✓ ½ cup plain peanut butter

Directions:

- ❖ Heat the heavy cream with the peanut butter, olive oil and erythritol in a small skillet over low heat without boiling for about 3 minutes. Remove from heat. In a bowl, beat egg yolks until creamy.

Ingredients:

- ✓ 1 tbsp olive oil
- ✓ 2 egg yolks
- ✓ ½ cup pecans, chopped

- ❖ Stir the eggs into the cream mixture. Continue stirring until a thick batter has formed, about 3 minutes. Pour the cream mixture into a bowl. Place in the refrigerator for 30 minutes. Stir in confectioners' sweetener.
- ❖ Pour mixture into ice cream maker and churn according to manufacturer's instructions. Stir in pecan later and spoon mixture into baking dish. Freeze for 2 hours before serving.

Nutrition: Calories 302, Fat 32g, Net Carbs 2g, Protein 5g

95) **Coffee Fat Bombs**

Preparation Time: 3 minutes + cooling time

Servings: 6

Ingredients:

- ✓ 6 tbsp prepared coffee at room temperature
- ✓ 1 ½ cups mascarpone cheese
- ✓ ½ cup melted butter

Directions:

- ❖ Beat mascarpone, butter, cocoa powder, erythritol and coffee with a hand mixer until creamy and fluffy, about 1 minute.

Ingredients:

- ✓ 3 tbsp unsweetened cocoa powder
- ✓ ¼ cup erythritol

- ❖ Fill muffin pans and freeze for 3 hours until firm.

Nutrition: Calories 145, fat 14g, net carbs 2g, protein 4g

96) **Mixed Berry and Mascarpone Bowl**

Preparation Time: 8 minutes

Servings: 4

Ingredients:

- ✓ 4 cups of Greek yogurt
- ✓ Liquid stevia to taste
- ✓ 1 ½ cups mascarpone cheese

Directions:

- ❖ Mix the yogurt, stevia and mascarpone in a bowl until evenly combined.

Ingredients:

- ✓ 1 ½ cups blueberries and raspberries
- ✓ 1 cup toasted pecans

- ❖ Divide the mixture among 4 bowls, divide the berries and pecans on top of the cream. Serve the dessert immediately.

Nutrition: Calories 480, Fat 40g, Net Carbs 5g, Protein 20g

97) Crazy Delicious Pudding

Preparation Time: 45 minutes   **Servings: 2**

Ingredients:

- ✓ 1 tangerine, sliced
- ✓ Juice of 2 tangerines
- ✓ 3 tbsp stevia
- ✓ 4 ounces of melted ghee
- ✓ ½ cup water

Directions:

- ❖ Grease a baking dish, arrange sliced tangerine on the bottom and set aside.
- ❖ In a bowl, mix ghee with stevia, flax meal, almonds, tangerine juice, flour and baking powder, stir and spread over tangerine slices.

Ingredients:

- ✓ 2 tbsp flax meal
- ✓ ¾ cup coconut flour
- ✓ 1 tsp baking powder
- ✓ ¾ cup almonds, ground
- ✓ Olive oil cooking spray
- ❖ Add the water to the Instant Pot, place the trivet on top, add the pan, cover and cook on high heat for 35 minutes.
- ❖ Set aside to cool, slice and serve.
- ❖ Enjoy!

Nutrition: Calories 200 | Fat: 2g | Carbohydrates: 3g | Protein: 4g | Fiber: 2g | Sugar: 0g

98) Wonderful berry pudding

Preparation Time: 45 minutes   **Servings: 2**

Ingredients:

- ✓ 1 cup almond flour
- ✓ 2 tbsp of lemon juice
- ✓ 2 cups blueberries
- ✓ 2 tbsp baking powder
- ✓ ½ tsp ground nutmeg
- ✓ ½ cup coconut milk
- ✓ 3 tbsp stevia

Directions:

- ❖ In a greased heatproof dish, mix blueberries and lemon juice, stir a little and spread over the bottom.
- ❖ In a bowl, mix flour with nutmeg, stevia, baking powder, vanilla, ghee, flaxseed meal, arrowroot and milk, mix well again and spread over blueberries.

Ingredients:

- ✓ 1 tbsp flax meal mixed with 1 tbsp water
- ✓ 3 tbsp melted ghee
- ✓ 1 tbsp vanilla extract
- ✓ 1 tbsp arrowroot powder
- ✓ 1 cup cold water

- ❖ Put the water in the Instant Pot, add the trivet and heatproof dish, cover and cook on high heat for 35 minutes.
- ❖ Let pudding cool, transfer to dessert bowls and serve.

Nutrition: Calories 220 | Fat: 4g | Carbohydrates: 9g | Protein: 6g | Fiber: 4g | Sugar: 2g

99) Orange Dessert

Preparation Time: 45 minutes

Servings: 2

Ingredients:

- ✓ 1 ¾ cups water
- ✓ 1 tsp baking powder
- ✓ 1 cup coconut flour
- ✓ 2 tbsp stevia
- ✓ ½ tbsp cinnamon powder
- ✓ 3 tbsp coconut oil, melted

Directions:

- ❖ In a bowl, mix flour with stevia, baking powder, cinnamon, 2 tbsp oil, milk, pecans and raisins; stir and transfer to a greased heatproof dish.
- ❖ Heat a small skillet over medium-high heat, mix ¾ cup water with the orange juice, orange zest and the rest of the oil, stir, bring to a boil and pour over the pecan mixture.

Ingredients:

- ✓ ½ cup coconut milk
- ✓ ½ cup pecans, chopped
- ✓ ½ cup raisins
- ✓ ½ cup orange peel, grated
- ✓ ¾ cup orange juice

- ❖ Place 1 cup of water in the Instant Pot, add the heatproof dish, cover and cook on High for 30 minutes.
- ❖ Serve cold.

Nutrition: Calories 142 | Fat: 3g | Carbohydrates: 3g | Protein: 3g | Fiber: 1g | Sugar: 1g

100) Great Pumpkin Dessert

Preparation Time: 40 minutes

Servings: 2

Ingredients:

- ✓ 1 and ½ tsp baking powder
- ✓ 2 cups of coconut flour
- ✓ ½ tsp baking soda
- ✓ ¼ tsp ground nutmeg
- ✓ 1 tsp cinnamon powder
- ✓ ¼ tsp ginger, grated
- ✓ 1 cup water

Directions:

- ❖ In a bowl, flour with baking powder, baking soda, cinnamon, ginger, nutmeg, oil, egg white, ghee, vanilla extract, pumpkin puree, stevia and lemon juice, mix well and transfer this to a greased cake pan.

Ingredients:

- ✓ 1 tbsp coconut oil, melted
- ✓ 1 egg white
- ✓ 1 tbsp vanilla extract
- ✓ 1 cup pumpkin puree
- ✓ 2 tbsp stevia
- ✓ 1 tbsp lemon juice

- ❖ Put the water in the Instant Pot, add the trivet, add the cake pan, cover and bake on High for 30 minutes.
- ❖ Allow cake to cool, cut and serve.

Nutrition: Calories 180 | Fat: 3g | Carbohydrates: 3g | Protein: 4g | Fiber: 2g | Sugar: 0g

101) Coconut cake with raspberries

Preparation Time: 30 min + cooling time

Servings: 8

Ingredients:

- ✓ 2 cups fresh raspberries
- ✓ 2 cups flaxseed meal
- ✓ 1 cup almond flour
- ✓ ½ cup melted butter

Directions:

- ❖ Preheat oven to 400 F. In a bowl, mix the flaxseed meal, almond flour and butter. Spread the mixture over the bottom of a baking dish. Bake for 20

Ingredients:

- ✓ 1 lemon, squeezed
- ✓ 1 cup coconut cream
- ✓ 1 cup coconut flakes
- ✓ 1 cup of whipping cream
- ❖ Carefully spread the coconut cream over the top, scatter with the coconut flakes and add the whipped cream over all. Garnish with remaining raspberries and chill in refrigerator for at least 2 hours.

minutes until the mixture is crispy. Allow to cool. In another bowl, mash 1 1/2 cups raspberries and stir in lemon juice. Spread the mixture over the crust.

Nutrition: Calories 413; Net carbs 5.4g; Fat 41g; Protein 7g

102)   Lemon Panna Cotta

Preparation Time: 30 minutes + cooling time

Ingredients:

- ✓ ½ cup coconut milk
- ✓ 1 cup heavy cream
- ✓ ¼ cup swerve sugar
- ✓ 5 tbsp unsweetened maple syrup

Directions:

- ❖ Heat the coconut milk and heavy cream in a saucepan over low heat. Add the swerve sugar, 3 tbsp maple syrup and 2 tbsp agar agar. Continue cooking for 3 minutes. Divide the mixture among 4 dessert cups and chill in the refrigerator for 5 hours. In a bowl, soak the remaining agar agar with hot water.

Ingredients:

- ✓ 3 tbsp agar agar
- ✓ ¼ cup hot water
- ✓ 3 tbsp water
- ✓ ½ lemon, squeezed
- ❖ Allow to bloom for 5 minutes. In a small saucepan, heat the water with the lemon juice. Stir in the remaining maple syrup and add the agar agar mixture. Whisk while cooking until no lumps form; let cool for 2 minutes. Remove cups, pour in mixture and refrigerate for 2 hours. When ready, remove cups, let stand for 15 minutes and serve.

Nutrition: Calories 208; Net carbs 2.8g; Fat 18g; Protein 2g

103)   Vanilla and Blackberry Sorbet

Preparation Time: 5 minutes

Ingredients:

- ✓ ¼ tsp vanilla extract
- ✓ 1 packet of gelatin
- ✓ 2 tbsp heavy whipping cream

Directions:

- ❖ Place gelatin in boiling water until dissolved. Place remaining ingredients in a blender and add gelatin.

Ingredients:

- ✓ 4 tbsp crushed blackberries
- ✓ 2 cups crushed ice
- ✓ 1 cup cold water
- ❖ Blend until smooth. Serve.

Nutrition: Calories 173; Net carbs 3.7g; Fat 10g; Protein 4g

104)   Flan with whipped cream

Preparation Time: 10 minutes + cooling time

Ingredients:

- ✓ ⅓ cup erythritol, for the caramel
- ✓ 2 cups almond milk
- ✓ 4 eggs
- ✓ 1 tbsp vanilla

Directions:

- ❖ Heat the erythritol for the caramel in a pan. Add 2-3 tbsp of water and bring to a boil. Reduce heat and cook until caramel turns golden brown. Carefully divide among 4 metal cups. Allow them to cool. In a bowl, mix the eggs, remaining erythritol, lemon zest and vanilla. Add the almond milk and beat again

Ingredients:

- ✓ 1 tbsp lemon zest
- ✓ ½ cup erythritol, for the custard
- ✓ 2 cups heavy whipping cream
- ✓ Mint leaves, for serving
- ❖ Pour enough hot water into the baking dish to halfway up the sides of the cups. Bake at 345 F for 45 minutes. Remove the ramekins and place them in the refrigerator for 4 hours. Take a knife and run slowly around the edges to spill onto plates. Serve with spoonfuls of cream and mint leaves.

until combined. Pour the cream into the caramel lined cups and place in a baking dish.

Nutrition: Calories 169; Net carbs 1.7g; Fat 10g; Protein 7g

105) **Chocolate and walnut cookies**

Preparation Time: 30 minutes

Servings: 4

Ingredients:
- ✓ 2/3 cup dark chocolate chips
- ✓ 4 ounces butter, softened
- ✓ 2 tbsp swerve sugar
- ✓ 2 tbsp brown sugar swerve
- ✓ 1 egg

Ingredients:
- ✓ 1 tsp vanilla extract
- ✓ ½ cup almond flour
- ✓ ½ tsp baking soda
- ✓ ½ cup chopped walnuts

Directions:
- ❖ Preheat oven to 350 F. In a bowl, beat butter, swerve sugar and swerve brown sugar until smooth. Beat in the egg and stir in the vanilla extract. In another bowl, combine the almond flour with the baking soda and mix into the wet ingredients. Add the chocolate chips and walnuts.

- ❖ Spoon full tbsp of batter onto a greased baking sheet, leaving 2 inches of space between each spoonful. Press each batter to flatten slightly. Bake for 15 minutes. Transfer to a rack to cool completely. Serve.

Nutrition: Calories 430; Net carbohydrates 3.5g; Fat 42g; Protein 6g

106) **Quick Blueberry Sorbet**

Preparation Time: 15 minutes + cooling time

Servings: 4

Ingredients:
- ✓ 4 cups frozen blueberries
- ✓ 1 cup sugar swerve

Ingredients:
- ✓ ½ lemon, squeezed
- ✓ ½ tsp salt
- ❖ Chill for 3 hours. Pour cooled juice into an ice cream maker and strain until mixture resembles ice cream. Spoon into a bowl and chill further for 3 hours.

Directions:
- ❖ In a blender, add blueberries, swerve, lemon juice and salt; process until smooth. Strain through a strainer into a bowl.

Nutrition: Calories 178; Net Carbs 2.3g; Fat 1g; Protein 0.6g

107) **Trifle of mixed berries**

Preparation Time: 3 minutes + cooling time

Servings: 4

Ingredients:
- ✓ ½ cup walnuts, toasted
- ✓ 1 avocado, chopped
- ✓ 1 cup mascarpone cheese, softened

Ingredients:
- ✓ 1 cup fresh blueberries
- ✓ 1 cup fresh raspberries
- ✓ 1 cup fresh blackberries
- ❖ Repeat the layering process a second time to finish the ingredients. Cover the glasses with plastic wrap and refrigerate for 45 minutes until fairly firm.

Directions:
- ❖ In four dessert glasses, divide half of the mascarpone, half of the berries (mixed), half of the walnuts and half of the avocado.

Nutrition: Calories 321, Fat 28.5g, Net Carbohydrates 8.3g, Protein 9.8g

108) Creamy Coconut Kiwi Drink

Preparation Time: 3 minutes

Servings: 4

Ingredients:
- ✓ 5 kiwis, picked pulp
- ✓ 2 tbsp of erythritol
- ✓ 2 cups unsweetened coconut milk

Directions:
- ❖ In a blender, process the kiwis, erythritol, milk, cream and ice cubes until smooth, about 3 minutes.

Ingredients:
- ✓ 2 cups of coconut cream
- ✓ 7 ice cubes
- ✓ Mint leaves for garnish
- ❖ Pour into four serving glasses, garnish with mint leaves and serve.

Nutrition: Calories 351, Fat 28g, Net Carbs 9.7g, Protein 16g

109) Walnut Cookies

Preparation Time: 15 minutes

Servings: 12

Ingredients:
- ✓ 1 egg
- ✓ 2 cups ground pecans
- ✓ ¼ cup sweetener

Directions:
- ❖ Preheat oven to 350°F. Mix ingredients, except walnuts, until combined. Make 20 balls with the dough and press them with your thumb onto a lined cookie sheet.

Ingredients:
- ✓ ½ tsp baking soda
- ✓ 1 tbsp butter
- ✓ 20 walnut halves
- ❖ Top each cookie with a walnut half. Bake for about 12 minutes.

Nutrition: Calories 101, Fat: 11g, Net Carbs: 0.6g, Protein: 1.6g

110) Chocolate Bark with Almonds

Preparation Time: 5 minutes + cooling time

Servings: 12

Ingredients:
- ✓ ½ cup toasted almonds, chopped
- ✓ ½ cup butter
- ✓ 10 drops of stevia

Directions:
- ❖ Melt the butter and chocolate together, in the microwave, for 90 seconds. Remove and stir in the stevia. Line a cookie sheet with wax paper and spread the chocolate evenly.

Ingredients:
- ✓ ¼ tsp salt
- ✓ ½ cup unsweetened coconut flakes
- ✓ 4 ounces dark chocolate
- ❖ Scatter the almonds on top, coconut flakes and sprinkle with salt. Place in the refrigerator for 1 hour.

Nutrition: Calories 161, Fat: 15.3g, Net Carbohydrates: 1.9g, Protein: 1.9g

111)   Raspberry Sorbet

Preparation Time: 10 minutes + cooling time

Servings: 1

Ingredients:
- ✓ ¼ tsp vanilla extract
- ✓ 1 package of gelatin, unsweetened
- ✓ 1 tbsp heavy whipping cream

Ingredients:
- ✓ 2 tbsp raspberry puree
- ✓ 1 ½ cups crushed ice

Directions:
- ❖ Cover gelatin with cold water in a small bowl. Allow to dissolve for 5 minutes. Transfer to a blender.

- ❖ Add remaining ingredients and ⅓ cup cold water. Blend until smooth and freeze for at least 2 hours.

Nutrition: Calories 173, Fat: 10g, Net Carbohydrates: 3.7g, Protein: 4g

112)   Coconut fat bombs

Preparation Time: 2 minutes + cooling time

Servings: 4

Ingredients:
- ✓ 2/3 cup coconut oil, melted
- ✓ 1 can of coconut milk (14 ounces)

Ingredients:
- ✓ 18 drops of liquid stevia
- ✓ 1 cup unsweetened coconut flakes
- ❖ Pour into silicone muffin molds and freeze for 1 hour to harden.

Directions:
- ❖ Mix the coconut oil with the milk and stevia. Stir in coconut flakes until well distributed.

Nutrition: Calories 214, fat 19g, net carbs 2g, protein 4g

113)   Dark Chocolate Mochaccino Ice Bombs

Preparation Time: 5 minutes + cooling time

Servings: 4

Ingredients:
- ✓ ½ pound of cream cheese
- ✓ 4 tbsp powdered sweetener
- ✓ 2 ounces of strong coffee

Ingredients:
- ✓ 2 tbsp unsweetened cocoa powder
- ✓ 1 tbsp cocoa butter, melted
- ✓ 2 1/2 ounces melted dark chocolate
- ❖ . Mix in the melted cocoa butter and chocolate and coat the bombs with it. Freeze for 2 hours.

Directions:
- ❖ Combine the cream cheese, sweetener, coffee and cocoa powder in a food processor. Spread 2 tbsp of the mixture and place on a lined tray.

Nutrition: Calories Calories 127, Fat: 13g, Net Carbohydrates: 1.4g, Protein: 1.9g

114)   Strawberry and ricotta parfait

Preparation Time: 10 minutes

Servings: 4

Ingredients:
- ✓ 2 cups strawberries, chopped
- ✓ 1 cup ricotta cheese

Ingredients:
- ✓ 2 tbsp sugar-free maple syrup
- ✓ 2 tbsp balsamic vinegar

Directions:
- ❖ Divide half of the strawberries among 4 small glasses and top with the ricotta.

- ❖ Drizzle with maple syrup, balsamic vinegar and finish with remaining strawberries. Serve.

Nutrition: Calories 164; Net carbs 3.1g; Fat 8.2g; Protein 7g

115) Creamy strawberry mousse

Preparation Time: 10 minutes + cooling time

Servings:

Ingredients:
- ✓ 2 cups frozen strawberries
- ✓ 2 tbsp sugar swerve

Directions:
- ❖ Pour 1 ½ cups of strawberries into a blender and process until smooth. Add the swerve sugar and process further. Pour in the egg whites and transfer the mixture to a bowl.

Ingredients:
- ✓ 1 large egg white
- ✓ 2 cups whipped cream
- ❖ Use an electric hand whisk to beat until the mixture is frothy. Pour mixture into dessert glasses and top with whipped cream and strawberries. Serve chilled.

Nutrition: Calories 145; Net carbohydrates 4.8g; Fat 6.8g; Protein 2g

116) Berry Clafoutis

Preparation Time: 45 minutes

Servings: 4

Ingredients:
- ✓ 4 eggs
- ✓ 2 tbsp coconut oil
- ✓ 2 cups berries
- ✓ 1 cup coconut milk

Directions:
- ❖ Preheat oven to 350 F. Place all ingredients except coconut oil, berries and sweetener powder in a blender until smooth.

Ingredients:
- ✓ 1 cup almond flour
- ✓ ¼ cup sweetener
- ✓ ½ tsp vanilla powder
- ✓ 1 tbsp powdered sweetener
- ❖ Gently add the berries. Grease a flan pan with coconut oil and pour in the mixture. Bake for 35 minutes. Sprinkle with powdered sugar and serve.

Nutrition: Calories 198; Net carbs 4.9g; Fat 16g; Protein 15g

117) Coconut and raspberry cheesecake

Preparation Time: 40 minutes + cooling time

Servings: 6

Ingredients:
- ✓ 2 egg whites
- ✓ 1 ¼ cups erythritol
- ✓ 3 cups desiccated coconut
- ✓ 1 tbsp coconut oil
- ✓ ¼ cup melted butter

Directions:
- ❖ Preheat oven to 350 F. Grease a baking sheet with coconut oil and line with baking paper. Mix egg whites, ¼ cup erythritol, coconut and butter until a crust forms and pour into the baking dish. Bake for 25 minutes. Allow to cool. Beat the cream cheese until smooth.

Ingredients:
- ✓ 3 tbsp lemon juice
- ✓ 6 ounces raspberries
- ✓ 1 cup whipped cream
- ✓ 3 tbsp lemon juice
- ✓ 24 ounces of cream cheese
- ❖ Add lemon juice and remaining erythritol. In another bowl, beat the heavy cream with an electric mixer. Fold the whipped cream into the cream cheese mixture; stir in the raspberries. Spread the filling over the baked crust. Refrigerate for 4 hours. Serve.

Nutrition: Calories 215; Net Carbs 3g; Fat 25g; Protein 5g

118) **Strawberry Chocolate Mousse**

Preparation Time: 30 minutes

Ingredients:
- ✓ 1 cup fresh strawberries, sliced
- ✓ 3 eggs
- ✓ 1 cup dark chocolate chips

Directions:
- ❖ Melt chocolate in a microwave-safe bowl in the microwave for 1 minute; let cool for 8 minutes. In a bowl, whip heavy cream until very smooth.

Servings: 4

Ingredients:
- ✓ 1 cup heavy cream
- ✓ 1 vanilla extract
- ✓ 1 tbsp sugar swerve
- ❖ Whisk in the eggs, vanilla extract and sugar swerve. Add the cooled chocolate. Divide the mousse between glasses, top with the strawberry and chill in the refrigerator. Serve.

Nutrition: Calories 400; Net Carbs 1.7g; Fat 25g; Protein 8g

119) **Peanut butter and chocolate ice cream bars**

Preparation Time: approxi 4 hours and 20 minutes

Ingredients:
- ✓ ¼ cup cocoa butter chunks, chopped
- ✓ 2 cups heavy whipping cream
- ✓ ⅔ cup peanut butter, softened
- ✓ 1 ½ cups almond milk

Directions:
- ❖ Mix the heavy cream, peanut butter, almond milk, vegetable glycerin and half of the xylitol until smooth. Place in an ice cream maker and follow instructions. Spread the ice cream into a lined baking dish and freeze for 4 hours.

Servings: 6

Ingredients:
- ✓ 1 tbsp vegetable glycerin
- ✓ 6 tbsp xylitol
- ✓ ¾ cup coconut oil
- ✓ 2 ounces unsweetened chocolate
- ❖ Mix coconut oil, cocoa butter, chocolate and remaining xylitol and microwave until melted; let cool slightly. Cut ice cream into bars. Dip into chocolate mixture. Serve.

Nutrition: Calories 345 Net carbohydrates 5g; Fat 32g; Protein 4g

120) **Lemon and yogurt mousse**

Preparation Time: 5 minutes + cooling time

Ingredients:
- ✓ 24 ounces plain yogurt, strained overnight in cheesecloth
- ✓ 2 cups powdered sugar swerve

Directions:
- ❖ Whip plain yogurt in a bowl with a hand mixer until light and fluffy. Stir in the swerve sugar, lemon juice and salt. Add the whipped cream to combine.

Servings:

Ingredients:
- ✓ 2 lemons, squeezed and peeled
- ✓ 1 cup whipped cream + extra for garnish
- ❖ Pour mousse into serving cups and refrigerate for 1 hour. Swirl with more whipped cream and garnish with lemon zest.

Nutrition: Calories 223; Net Carbs 3g; Fat 18g; Protein 12g

PART II: INTRODUCTION

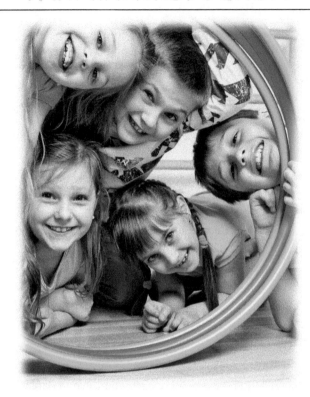

As a parent, hearing the words "diet for kids" may sound a little strange unless your child suffers from obesity. His pediatrician has recommended that he lose weight to avoid the risk of developing chronic conditions. Another possible scenario that could lead to this is if you and your partner follow the same diet or lifestyle. For example, if you are vegan, there is a high possibility that you will also raise your children as vegans. Aside from the reasons above, you may not see the essence of putting your child on a specific diet.

I can vividly recall the instance when I decided to put my children on this diet. I had been following Paleo religiously for about a year and had personally experienced the many benefits of the diet. I discovered that Paleo is one of the diets that children can follow, to my surprise and delight. It provides several health benefits for children as well.

Although food, mainly processed food, is readily available today, our early ancestors did not have access to the variety of options we have now. The foods our ancestors ate depended on their geographic conditions, the paleontological period in which they lived, and changes in the seasons. In other words, they barely had a choice - they ate only what was hunted and gathered from their environment. If they couldn't find food, they didn't eat. Despite this, our early ancestors never had to deal with as many diet-related health problems as we face today.

Nowadays, our children eat everything and whenever they want. They have gotten so used to having food at their fingertips that they barely think about the importance of eating healthy.

The Paleo diet consists of completely healthy foods like grass-fed meats, seafood, poultry, healthy oils, seeds, and nuts. With this diet, your kids will lose their uncontrollable cravings for processed and refined foods, as well as trans fats. Paleo is one of the most popular diets these days, and for a good reason. I've experienced several health benefits by sticking to this diet, such as overcoming prediabetes, brain fog, and bloating. I've also lost my excess weight! With this diet, my children and I also enjoy stable energy levels, we sleep better, our skin and hair are healthier, and we've noticed an overall improvement in our mood. Later, we'll discuss these health benefits in more detail to give you a better idea of what you and your kids should potentially expect by following this diet.

If you're a mom like me (or a dad) and you're thinking about trying Paleo, or you're already following this diet, you may also be thinking about putting your kids on Paleo. Therefore, you want to learn everything you can about Paleo for kids before you start. This is a significant first step. Educating yourself about this diet, its benefits, and how you can safely introduce it to your kids are essential steps to help you find success.

Here's another great thing about Paleo that I discovered while doing my research: according to one study, following this approach for a few days can grant you several health benefits, such as improved glucose tolerance, blood pressure, and insulin sensitivity (Frasetto et al., 2011). The same study also showed improvements in the metabolism and circulatory system of most participants.

Once you know more about Paleo, the next thing you need to think about is how to overcome the challenge of introducing this particular diet to your children. The Paleo diet is very different from the standard American diet, or the "traditional diet" that requires no rules. When introducing this diet to your children, try to think about how you would introduce a new set of rules or skills to them. Start slowly, be patient, and don't expect your children to get used to it right away. Here are some tips for getting started:

Try to find healthier alternatives for their favorite foods. This will make the transition to the Paleo diet easier.

Learn how to cook their meals and snacks, so they get used to the diet at school as well.

Add a new food to their menu every day. Avoid overwhelming your children by serving meals where everything is new. When you introduce something new, encourage them to try it.

If your children refuse to try a new type of food, avoid forcing it on them. Instead, leave it alone.

Consider involving your children in the preparation and cooking of meals. These tasks are fun, educational and can help your children learn to be more open to trying new foods.

At some point, you will need to stop preparing separate meals for your children. This is the time when you can start enjoying Paleo as a family. However, keep a side dish or dessert familiar to your children so that they still feel like they have a choice.

It is also essential that you talk about this new diet change with your children. The conversation you have with your children about Paleo depends on the age they are. Why not try a story about cave dwellers and how they ate? Then you can use it as a gateway to present your plans to start following Paleo. If you have an older child, one who already understands the concept of health, then dive right into explaining to them the benefits of this diet.

Just avoid delving into technical or scientific explanations of the benefits. Make sure your answers are age-appropriate to make sure your kids understand why you want them to start following Paleo. Communicating with your children in this way can make the whole journey much easier and positive for both parties.

As a parent interested in Paleo for kids, you will benefit immensely from this book. Here you will learn more about Paleo and what it entails. I will share tips on discussing food and nutrition with your children, how to get your family members involved in going Paleo, and how to keep this diet together. I will also share several easy and affordable recipes for you to cook in the comfort of your own home. Learning how to cook for your kids is one of the most effective ways to follow Paleo in the long run.

Since you already know your children's current diet and eating habits, learning all you can about Paleo will help you make smarter, healthier choices for them. You'll also gain valuable insights into the essential components of making any meal more Paleo-friendly and how to adjust your approach to suit your family's needs.

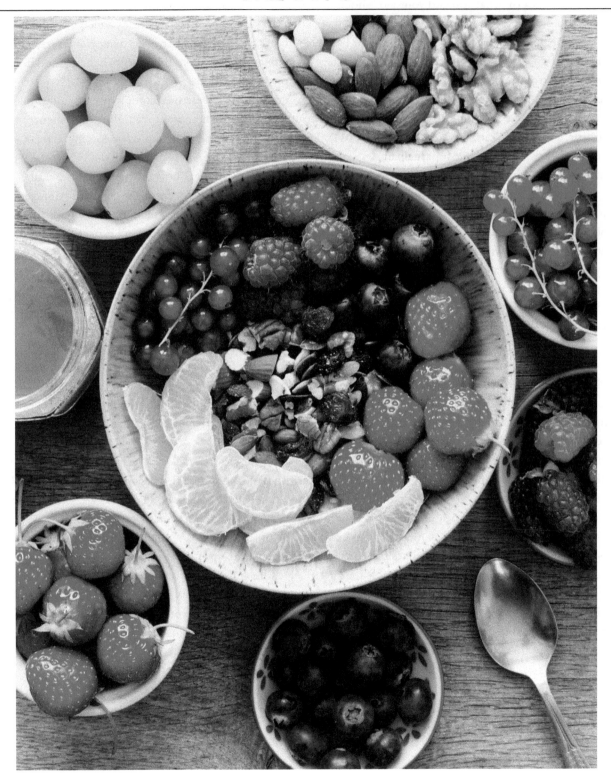

121) **Tropical Coconut Flour Bagels**

Preparation Time: 25 minutes

Servings: 6

Ingredients:

- ✓ ½ cup coconut flour
- ✓ 6 eggs, beaten in a bowl
- ✓ ½ cup vegetable broth
- ✓ ¼ cup flaxseed meal

Ingredients:

- ✓ 1 tsp onion powder
- ✓ 1 tsp dried parsley
- ✓ 1 tsp chia seeds
- ✓ 1 tsp sesame seeds
- ✓ 1 onion, chopped
- ❖ Top with onion and sprinkle with chia and sesame seeds. Bake the bagels for 20 minutes. Remove and let cool before serving.

Directions:

- ❖ Preheat oven to 350°F. Mix the coconut flour, eggs, vegetable broth, flaxseed meal, onion powder, and parsley in a bowl and stir well. Spoon the mixture into a donut tray

Nutrition: Calories 426, Fat 19.1g, Net Carbs 0.4g, Protein 33.1g

122) **Spanish Chorizo and Mozzarella Omelet**

Preparation Time: 15 minutes

Servings: 2

Ingredients:

- ✓ 4 eggs
- ✓ 2 oz mozzarella cheese, sliced
- ✓ 1 tbsp butter

Directions:

- ❖ Whisk the eggs with salt and pepper in a bowl. Melt the butter in a skillet over medium heat. Pour the eggs and cook for 1 minute. Top with the chorizo. Arrange the tomato and mozzarella over the chorizo.

Ingredients:

- ✓ 4 thin chorizo slices
- ✓ 1 tomato, sliced
- ✓ Salt and black pepper to taste
- ❖ Cover the skillet and cook for about 3-5 minutes until the omelet is set. Remove the pan from the heat. Run a spatula around the omelet's edges and flip it onto a plate, folded side down. Serve with salad.

Nutrition: Calories 451, Fat: 36.5g, Net Carbs: 3g, Protein: 30g

123) **Italian-style Sausage Stacks**

Preparation Time: 20 minutes

Servings: 6

Ingredients:

- ✓ 6 Italian sausage patties
- ✓ 4 tbsp olive oil
- ✓ 2 ripe avocados, pitted

Directions:

- ❖ In a skillet, warm the oil over medium heat and fry the sausage patties about 8 minutes until lightly browned and firm. Remove the patties to a plate. Spoon the avocado into a bowl and mash it with a fork. Season with salt and black pepper. Spread the mash on the sausages.

Ingredients:

- ✓ Salt and black pepper to taste
- ✓ 6 fresh eggs
- ✓ Red pepper flakes to garnish
- ❖ Boil 3 cups of water in a wide pan over high heat and reduce to simmer (don't boil). Crack each egg into a small bowl and gently put the egg into the simmering water. Poach for 2-3 minutes. Use a perforated spoon to remove from the water on a paper towel to dry. Repeat with the other 5 eggs. Top each stack with a poached egg and sprinkle with chili flakes. Serve with turnip wedges.

Nutrition: Calories 378, Fat 23g, Net Carbs 5g, Protein 16g

124) **Paleo Eggs and Crabmeat with Creme Fraiche Salsa**

Preparation Time: 15 minutes

Servings: 3

Ingredients:
- ✓ 1 tbsp olive oil
- ✓ 6 eggs, whisked
- ✓ 1 (6 oz) can crabmeat, flaked
- ✓ Salsa
- ✓ ¾ cup crème fraiche

Directions:
- ❖ Warm the olive oil a pan over medium heat. Add in the eggs and scramble them. Stir in crabmeat and season with salt and pepper. Cook until cooked thoroughly. In a dish, combine all salsa ingredients

Ingredients:
- ✓ ½ cup scallions, chopped
- ✓ ½ tsp garlic powder
- ✓ Salt and black pepper to taste
- ✓ ½ tsp fresh dill, chopped

- ❖ . Split the egg/crabmeat mixture among serving plates. Serve alongside the scallions and salsa to the side.

Nutrition: Calories 334; Fat: 26.2g, Net Carbs: 4.4g, Protein: 21.1g

125) **Easy Cheese and Aioli Eggs**

Preparation Time: 20 minutes

Servings: 4

Ingredients:
- ✓ 4 eggs, hard-boiled and chopped
- ✓ 14 oz tuna in brine, drained
- ✓ ¼ lettuce head, torn into pieces
- ✓ 2 green onions, finely chopped
- ✓ ½ cup feta cheese, crumbled

Directions:
- ❖ Set the eggs in a serving bowl. Place in tuna, onion, feta cheese, lettuce, and sour cream. In a bowl, mix the mayonnaise, lemon juice, and garlic

Ingredients:
- ✓ ⅓ cup sour cream
- ✓ Aioli
- ✓ 1 cup mayonnaise
- ✓ 2 cloves garlic, minced
- ✓ 1 tbsp lemon juice
- ✓ Salt and black pepper to taste
- ❖ Season with salt and pepper. Pour the aioli into the serving bowl and stir to incorporate everything. Serve with pickles.

Nutrition: Calories 355; Fat 22.5g, Net Carbs 1.8g, Protein 29.5g

126) **Special Kielbasa and Roquefort Waffles**

Preparation Time: 20 minutes

Servings: 2

Ingredients:
- ✓ ½ tsp parsley, chopped
- ✓ ½ tsp chili pepper flakes
- ✓ 4 eggs

Directions:
- ❖ In a bowl, combine all ingredients except chives. Preheat the waffle iron. Pour in some batter and close the lid

Ingredients:
- ✓ ½ cup Roquefort cheese, crumbled
- ✓ 4 slices kielbasa, chopped
- ✓ 2 tbsp fresh chives, chopped
- ❖ Cook for 5 minutes until golden brown. Repeat with the rest of the batter. Decorate with chives.

Nutrition: Calories 470; Fat: 40.3g, Net Carbs: 2.9g, Protein: 24.4g

127)   **Rich Baked Quail Eggs in Avocados**

Preparation Time: 15 minutes   Servings: 4

Ingredients:

✓ 2 large avocados, halved and pitted
✓ 4 small eggs

Ingredients:

✓ Salt and black pepper to taste

Directions:

❖ Preheat oven to 400°F. Crack the quail eggs into the avocado halves and place them on a greased baking sheet.

❖ Bake the filled avocados in the oven for 8-10 minutes until eggs are cooked. Season and serve.

Nutrition: Calories 234, Fat 19.1g, Net Carbs 2.2g, Protein 8.2g

128)   **Italian-style Fontina Cheese and Chorizo Waffles**

Preparation Time: 30 minutes   Servings: 6

Ingredients:

✓ 6 eggs
✓ 2 tbsp butter, melted
✓ 1 cup almond flour

Ingredients:

✓ Salt and black pepper to taste
✓ 3 chorizo sausages, cooked, chopped
✓ 1 cup fontina cheese, shredded
❖ Preheat the waffle iron and grease it with cooking spray. Pour in the egg mixture and cook for 5 minutes until golden brown. Serve hot.

Directions:

❖ In a shallow bowl, beat the eggs with salt and pepper. Add in the almond milk, butter, fontina cheese, and sausages and stir to combine. Let it sit for 15-20 minutes

Nutrition: Calories 316; Fat: 25g, Net Carbs: 1.5g, Protein: 20.2g

129)   **Tropical Coconut Porridge with Strawberries**

Preparation Time: approx. 12 minutes   Servings: 2

Ingredients:

✓ Flax egg: 1 tbsp flax seed powder + 3 tbsp water
✓ 1 oz olive oil
✓ 1 tbsp coconut flour

Ingredients:

✓ 1 pinch ground chia seeds
✓ 5 tbsp coconut cream
✓ 1 pinch salt
✓ Strawberries to serve
❖ Cook, while stirring continuously until the desired consistency is achieved. Top with strawberries.

Directions:

❖ For flax egg, in a bowl, mix flax seed powder with water, and let soak for 5 minutes. Place a saucepan over low heat and pour in olive oil, flax egg, flour, chia, coconut cream, and salt.

Nutrition: Calories 521; Net Carbs 4g; Fat 49g; Protein 10g

130) Original Mexican Tofu Scramble

Preparation Time: approx. 45 minutes

Servings: 4

Ingredients:
- ✓ 8 oz tofu, scrambled
- ✓ 2 tbsp butter
- ✓ 1 green bell pepper, chopped
- ✓ 1 tomato, finely chopped

Directions:
- ❖ Melt butter in a skillet over medium heat. Fry the tofu until golden brown, stirring occasionally, about 5 minutes.

Ingredients:
- ✓ 2 tbsp chopped scallions
- ✓ Salt and black pepper to taste
- ✓ 1 tsp Mexican chili powder
- ✓ 3 oz grated Parmesan cheese
- ❖ . Stir in bell pepper, tomato, scallions, and cook until the vegetables are soft, 4 minutes. Season with salt, pepper, chili powder and stir in Parmesan cheese, about 2 minutes. Spoon the scramble into a serving platter and serve warm.

Nutrition: Calories254; Net Carbs 3g; Fat 19g; Protein 16g

131) Special No-Bread Avocado Sandwiches

Preparation Time: approx. 10 minutes

Servings: 2

Ingredients:
- ✓ 1 avocado, sliced
- ✓ 1 large red tomato, sliced
- ✓ 4 little gem lettuce leaves

Directions:
- ❖ Arrange the lettuce on a flat serving plate. Smear each leave with butter and arrange tofu slices on the leaves

Ingredients:
- ✓ ½ oz butter, softened
- ✓ 4 tofu slices
- ✓ 1 tsp chopped parsley
- ❖ Top with the avocado and tomato slices. Garnish the sandwiches with parsley and serve.

Nutrition: Calories 385; Net Carbs 4g; Fat 32g; Protein 12g

132) Easy Blueberry Chia Pudding

Preparation Time:approx. 10 min + chilling time

Servings: 2

Ingredients:
- ✓ ¾ cup coconut milk
- ✓ ½ tsp vanilla extract
- ✓ ½ cup blueberries

Directions:
- ❖ In a blender, pour coconut milk, vanilla extract, and half of the blueberries. Process the ingredients in high speed until the blueberries have incorporated into the liquid

Ingredients:
- ✓ 2 tbsp chia seeds
- ✓ 1 tbsp chopped walnuts

- ❖ . Mix in chia seeds. Share the mixture into 2 breakfast jars, cover, and refrigerate for 4 hours to allow it to gel. Garnish with the remaining blueberries and walnuts. Serve.

Nutrition: Calories 301; Net Carbs 6g; Fat 23g; Protein 9g

133) Easy Creamy Sesame Bread

Preparation Time: approx. 40 minutes

Servings: 6

Ingredients:
- ✓ 4 tbsp flax seed powder
- ✓ 1 cup cream cheese
- ✓ 5 tbsp sesame oil
- ✓ 1 cup coconut flour

Ingredients:
- ✓ 2 tbsp psyllium husk powder
- ✓ 1 tsp salt
- ✓ 1 tsp baking powder
- ✓ 1 tbsp sesame seeds
- ❖ Spread the dough in a greased baking tray. Allow to stand for 5 minutes and then brush with remaining sesame oil. Sprinkle with sesame seeds and bake the dough for 30 minutes. Slice and serve.

Directions:
- ❖ In a bowl, mix flax seed powder with 1 ½ cups water until smoothly combined and set aside to soak for 5 minutes. Preheat oven to 400 F. When the flax egg is ready, beat in cream cheese and 4 tbsp sesame oil until mixed. Whisk in coconut flour, psyllium husk powder, salt, and baking powder until adequately blended

Nutrition: Calories 285; Net Carbs 1g; Fat 26g; Protein 8g

134) Special Bulletproof Coffee

Preparation Time: approx. 3 minutes

Servings: 2

Ingredients:
- ✓ 2 ½ heaping tbsp ground bulletproof coffee beans
- ✓ 1 tbsp coconut oil

Ingredients:
- ✓ 2 tbsp unsalted butter

- ❖ Blend the mixture until frothy and smooth.

Directions:
- ❖ Using a coffee maker, brew one cup of coffee with the ground coffee beans and 1 cup of water. Transfer the coffee to a blender and add the coconut oil and butter

Nutrition: Calories 336; Net Carbs 0g; Fat 36g; Protein 2g

135) Easy Breakfast Naan Bread

Preparation Time: approx. 25 minutes

Servings: 6

Ingredients:
- ✓ ¾ cup almond flour
- ✓ 2 tbsp psyllium husk powder
- ✓ 1 tsp salt
- ✓ ½ tsp baking powder

Ingredients:
- ✓ ¼ cup olive oil
- ✓ 2 cups boiling water
- ✓ 8 oz butter
- ✓ 2 garlic cloves, minced
- ❖ . Melt half of the butter in a frying pan over medium heat and fry the naan on both sides to have a golden color. Transfer to a plate and keep warm. Add the remaining butter to the pan and sauté garlic until fragrant, about 1 minute. Pour the garlic butter into a bowl and serve as a dip along with the naan.

Directions:
- ❖ In a bowl, mix almond flour, psyllium husk powder, ½ tsp of salt, and baking powder. Mix in olive oil and boiling water to combine the ingredients like a thick porridge. Stir and allow the dough rise for 5 minutes. Divide the dough into 6 pieces and mold into balls. Place the balls on a parchment paper and flatten

Nutrition: Calories 224; Net Carbs 3g; Fat 19g; Protein 4g

136)   Italian Mascarpone Snapped Amaretti Biscuits

Preparation Time: 25 minutes

Ingredients:
- ✓ 6 egg whites
- ✓ 1 egg yolk, beaten
- ✓ 1 tsp vanilla bean paste
- ✓ 4 tbsp swerve sugar
- ✓ A pinch of salt
- ✓ ¼ cup ground fragrant almonds

Directions:
- ❖ Preheat oven to 300°F. Line a baking sheet with parchment paper. In a bowl, beat egg whites, salt, and vanilla paste with a hand mixer while you gradually spoon in the swerve sugar until stiff. Add in almonds and fold in the egg yolk, lemon juice, and amaretto liquor. Spoon mixture into a piping bag.
- ❖ Press out 50 mounds on the baking sheet. Bake the biscuits for 15 minutes until golden brown.

Nutrition: Calories 165, Fat 13g, Net Carbs 3g, Protein 9g

Servings: 6

Ingredients:
- ✓ 1 lemon juice
- ✓ 7 tbsp sugar-free amaretto liquor
- ✓ ¼ cup mascarpone cheese
- ✓ ¼ cup butter, room temperature
- ✓ ¾ cup swerve confectioner's sugar

- ❖ Transfer to a wire rack to cool. Whisk the mascarpone cheese, butter, and swerve confectioner's sugar with the cleaned electric mixer. Spread a scoop of mascarpone cream onto the case of half of the biscuits and snap with the remaining biscuits. Dust with some swerve confectioner's sugar and serve.

137)   Special Turkey Sausage Egg Cups

Preparation Time: 15 minutes

Ingredients:
- ✓ 2 tsp butter
- ✓ 8 eggs, beaten
- ✓ Salt and black pepper to taste

Directions:
- ❖ Preheat oven to 400°F. Melt butter in a skillet over medium heat. Cook the turkey sausages for 4-5 minutes. In a bowl, mix 4 eggs, sausages, cheese, and seasonings.

Nutrition: Calories 423; Fat: 34.1g, Net Carbs: 2.2g, Protein: 26.5g

Servings: 4

Ingredients:
- ✓ ½ tsp dried rosemary
- ✓ 1 cup pecorino romano, grated
- ✓ 4 turkey sausages, chopped
- ❖ Divide between greased muffin cups and bake for 4 minutes. Crack an egg into the middle of each cup. Bake for 4 more minutes. Serve cooled.

138)   Easy Cheese Stuffed Avocados

Preparation Time: 20 minutes

Ingredients:
- ✓ 3 avocados, halved, pitted, skin on
- ✓ ½ cup feta cheese, crumbled
- ✓ ½ cup cheddar cheese, grated

Directions:
- ❖ Preheat oven to 360°F. Lay avocado halves in a baking dish. In a bowl, mix both types of cheeses, pepper, eggs, and salt

Nutrition: Calories 342; Fat: 30.4g, Net Carbs: 7.5g, Protein: 11.1g

Servings: 4

Ingredients:
- ✓ 2 eggs, beaten
- ✓ Salt and black pepper to taste
- ✓ 1 tbsp fresh basil, chopped
- ❖ Split the mixture into the avocado halves. Bake for 15 minutes. Top with basil and serve.

139) Special Duo-Cheese Omelet with Pimenta and Basil

Preparation Time: 15 minutes

Servings: 2

Ingredients:
- ✓ 1 tbsp olive oil
- ✓ 4 eggs, beaten
- ✓ Salt and black pepper to taste
- ✓ ¼ tsp paprika

Directions:
- ❖ Warm the olive oil in a pan over medium. Season the eggs with cayenne pepper, salt, paprika, and pepper. Transfer to the pan and ensure they are evenly spread. Cook for 5 minutes

Ingredients:
- ✓ ¼ tsp cayenne pepper
- ✓ ½ cup asiago cheese, shredded
- ✓ ½ cup cheddar cheese, shredded
- ✓ 2 tbsp fresh basil, roughly chopped
- ❖ Top with the asiago and cheddar cheeses. Slice the omelet into two halves. Decorate with fresh basil and serve.

Nutrition: Calories 490; Fat: 44.6g, Net Carbs: 4.5g, Protein: 22.7g

140) Easy and Quick Blue Cheese Omelet

Preparation Time: 15 minutes

Servings: 2

Ingredients:
- ✓ 4 eggs
- ✓ Salt to taste
- ✓ 1 tbsp sesame oil

Directions:
- ❖ In a bowl, beat the eggs with salt. Warm the oil in a pan over medium heat. Add in the eggs and cook as you swirl the eggs around the pan.

Ingredients:
- ✓ ½ cup blue cheese, crumbled
- ✓ 1 tomato, thinly sliced

- ❖ Cook eggs until set. Top with cheese. Decorate with tomato and serve.

Nutrition: Calories 307Calories; Fat: 25g, Net Carbs: 2.5g, Protein: 18.5g

141) Tropical Coconut and Walnut Chia Pudding

Preparation Time: 10 minutes

Servings: 1

Ingredients:
- ✓ ½ tsp vanilla extract
- ✓ ½ cup water
- ✓ 1 tbsp chia seeds
- ✓ 2 tbsp hemp seeds
- ✓ 1 tbsp flaxseed meal

Directions:
- ❖ Put chia seeds, hemp seeds, flaxseed meal, almond meal, stevia, and coconut in a saucepan and pour over the water. Simmer over medium heat, occasionally stirring until creamed and thickened, about 3-4 minutes

Ingredients:
- ✓ 2 tbsp almond meal
- ✓ 2 tbsp shredded coconut
- ✓ ¼ tsp granulated stevia
- ✓ 1 tbsp walnuts, chopped

- ❖ Stir in vanilla. When it is ready, spoon into a serving bowl, sprinkle with walnuts, and serve.

Nutrition: Calories Calories 334, Fat: 29g, Net Carbs: 1.5g Protein: 15g

142) **Italian Cheese Ciabatta with Pepperoni**

Preparation Time: 30 minutes

Servings: 6

Ingredients:

- ✓ 10 oz cream cheese, melted
- ✓ 2 ½ cups mozzarella, shredded
- ✓ 4 large eggs, beaten
- ✓ 3 tbsp Romano cheese, grated

Directions:

- ❖ In a bowl, combine eggs, mozzarella cheese, cream cheese, baking powder, pork rinds, and Romano cheese. Form into 6 chiabatta shapes

Ingredients:

- ✓ ½ cup pork rinds, crushed
- ✓ 2 tsp baking powder
- ✓ ½ cup tomato puree
- ✓ 12 pepperoni slices
- ❖ Set a pan over medium heat. Cook each ciabatta for 2 minutes per side. Sprinkle tomato puree over each one and top with pepperoni slices to serve.

Nutrition: Calories Calories 464, Fat: 33.6g, Net Carbs: 9.1g, Protein: 31.1g

143) **Special Seed Breakfast Loaf**

Preparation Time: approx. 55 minutes

Servings: 6

Ingredients:

- ✓ ¾ cup coconut flour
- ✓ 1 cup almond flour
- ✓ 3 tbsp baking powder
- ✓ 2 tbsp psyllium husk powder
- ✓ 2 tbsp desiccated coconut
- ✓ 5 tbsp sesame seeds
- ✓ ¼ cup flaxseed
- ✓ ¼ cup hemp seeds

Directions:

- ❖ Preheat oven to 350 F. In a bowl, mix coconut and almond flours, baking powder, psyllium husk, desiccated coconut, sesame seeds, flaxseed, hemp seeds, ground caraway and poppy seeds, salt, and allspice

Ingredients:

- ✓ 1 tsp ground caraway seeds
- ✓ 1 tbsp poppy seeds
- ✓ 1 tsp salt
- ✓ 1 tsp allspice
- ✓ 6 eggs
- ✓ 1 cup cream cheese, softened
- ✓ ¾ cup heavy cream
- ✓ 4 tbsp sesame oil
- ❖ In another bowl, whisk eggs, cream cheese, heavy cream, and sesame oil. Pour the mixture into the dry ingredients and combine both into a smooth dough. Pour the dough in a greased loaf pan. Bake for 45 minutes. Remove onto a rack and let cool.

Nutrition: Calories 584; Net Carbs 7.4g; Fat 50g; Protein 23g

144) Everyday Blackberry Chia Pudding

Preparation Time: approx. 45 minutes

Servings: 4

Ingredients:

- ✓ 1 ½ cups coconut milk
- ✓ ½ cup Greek yogurt
- ✓ 4 tsp sugar-free maple syrup
- ✓ 1 tsp vanilla extract
- ✓ 7 tbsp chia seeds

Ingredients:

- ✓ 1 cup fresh blackberries
- ✓ 3 tbsp chopped almonds
- ✓ Mint leaves to garnish

Directions:

- ❖ In a bowl, combine coconut milk, Greek yogurt, sugar-free maple syrup, and vanilla extract until evenly combined. Mix in the chia seeds. Puree half of blackberries in a bowl using a fork and stir in the yogurt mixture

- ❖ . Share the mixture into medium mason jars, cover the lids and refrigerate for 30 minutes to thicken the pudding. Remove the jars, take off the lid, and stir the mixture. Garnish with remaining blackberries, almonds, and some mint leaves.

Nutrition: Calories 309; Net Carbs 6.8g; Fat 26g; Protein 7g

145) Easy Blueberry Soufflé

Preparation Time: approx. 35 minutes

Servings: 4

Ingredients:

- ✓ 1 cup frozen blueberries
- ✓ 5 tbsp erythritol
- ✓ 4 egg yolks

Ingredients:

- ✓ 3 egg whites
- ✓ 1 tsp olive oil
- ✓ ½ lemon, zested
- ❖ Fold egg white mixture into egg yolk mix. Heat olive oil in a pan over low heat. Add in olive oil and pour in the egg mixture; swirl to spread. Cook for 3 minutes and transfer to the oven; bake for 2-3 minutes or until puffed and set. Plate soufflé and spoon blueberry sauce all over. Garnish with lemon zest.

Directions:

- ❖ Pour blueberries, 2 tbsp erythritol and 1 tbsp water in a saucepan. Cook until the berries soften and become syrupy, 8-10 minutes. Set aside. Preheat oven to 350 F. In a bowl, beat egg yolks and 1 tbsp of erythritol until thick and pale. In another bowl, whisk egg whites until foamy. Add in remaining erythritol and whisk until soft peak forms, 3-4 minutes.

Nutrition: Calories 99; Net Carbs 2.8g; Fat 5.9g; Protein 5.5g

146) American Cheddar Biscuits

Preparation Time: approx. 30 minutes

Servings: 4

Ingredients:

- ✓ 2 ½ cups almond flour
- ✓ 2 tsp baking powder
- ✓ 2 eggs beaten

Ingredients:

- ✓ 3 tbsp melted butter
- ✓ ¾ cup grated cheddar cheese

- ❖ Mold 12 balls out of the mixture and arrange on the sheet at 2-inch intervals. Bake for 25 minutes until golden brown. Remove, let cool, and serve.

Directions:

- ❖ Preheat oven to 350 F. Line a baking sheet with parchment paper. In a bowl, mix flour, baking powder, and eggs until smooth. Whisk in the melted butter and cheddar cheese until well combined.

Nutrition: Calories 355; Net Carbs 1.4g; Fat 28g, Protein 21g

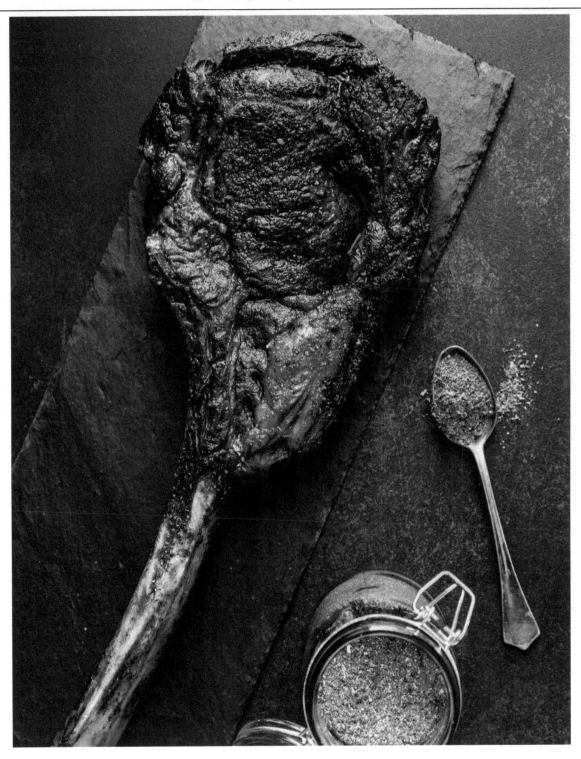

147) **Easy Paleo Shrimp Burgers**

Preparation Time: 30 minutes   **Servings: 4**

Ingredients:

✓ 2 tbsp. cilantro, chopped
✓ 1 and ½ pounds shrimp, peeled and deveined
✓ 2 tbsp. chives, chopped
✓ Salt and pepper to aste
✓ 1 garlic clove, minced
✓ ¼ cup radishes, minced
✓ 1 tsp. lemon zest
✓ ¼ cup celery, minced
✓ 1 egg, whisked
✓ 1 tbsp. lemon juice

Ingredients:

✓ ¼ cup almond meal
✓ For the salsa:
✓ · 1 avocado, pitted, peeled and chopped
✓ · 1 cup pineapple, chopped
✓ · 2 tbsp. red onion, chopped
✓ · ¼ cup bell peppers, chopped
✓ · 1 tbsp. lime juice
✓ · 1 tbsp. cilantro, finely chopped
✓ · Salt and black pepper to taste

Directions:

❖ In a bowl, mix pineapple with avocado, bell peppers, two tbsp red onion, one tbsp lime juice, salt, pepper to the taste and one tbsp cilantro, stir well and keep in the fridge for now.

❖ In your food processor, mix shrimp with two tbsp cilantro, chives, and garlic and blend well.

❖ Transfer to a bowl and mix with radishes, celery, lemon zest, lemon juice, egg, almond meal, salt, and pepper to the taste and stir well.

❖ Shape 4 burgers, place them on preheated grill over medium-high heat and cook for 5 minutes on each side.

❖ Divide shrimp burgers between plates and serve with the salsa you've made earlier on the side.

❖ Enjoy!

Nutrition: Calories 238 | Fat: 12g | Carbs: 13g | Protein: 15g | Fiber: 3g | Sugar: 0g

148) **Lovely Paleo Scallops Tartar**

Preparation Time: 15 minutes   **Servings: 2**

Ingredients:

✓ 6 scallops, diced
✓ Salt and pepper to taste
✓ 3 strawberries, chopped
✓ 1 tbsp. extra virgin olive oil

Ingredients:

✓ 1 tbsp. green onions, minced
✓ Juice of ½ lemon
✓ ½ tbsp. basil leaves, finely chopped

Directions:

❖ In a bowl, mix strawberries with scallops, basil, and onions and stir well.

❖ Add olive oil, salt, pepper to the taste and lemon juice and stir well again.

❖ Keep in the fridge until you serve.

❖ Enjoy!

Nutrition: Calories 180 | Fat: 27g | Carbs: 3g | Protein: 24g | Fiber: 0g | Sugar: 0g

149) **Tasty Paleo Shrimp Skewers**

Preparation Time: 20 minutes   **Servings: 4**

Ingredients:

- ✓ ½ lb. sausages, chopped and already cooked
- ✓ ½ lb. shrimp, peeled and deveined
- ✓ 2 tbsp. extra virgin olive oil
- ✓ 2 zucchinis, cubed
- ✓ Salt and black pepper to taste
- ✓ For the Creole seasoning:

Directions:

- ❖ In a bowl, mix paprika with garlic powder, onion one, chili powder, oregano, and thyme and stir well.
- ❖ In another bowl, combine shrimp with sausage, zucchini, and oil and toss to coat.
- ❖ Pour paprika mix over shrimp mix and stir well.

Ingredients:

- ✓ ½ tbsp. garlic powder
- ✓ 2 tbsp. paprika
- ✓ ½ tbsp. onion powder
- ✓ ¼ tbsp. oregano, dried
- ✓ ½ tbsp. chili powder
- ✓ ¼ tbsp. thyme, dried
- ❖ Arrange sausage, shrimp, and zucchini on skewers alternating pieces, place them on preheated grill over medium-high heat and cook for 8 minutes, flipping skewers from time to time.
- ❖ Arrange on a platter and serve.
- ❖ Enjoy!

Nutrition: Calories 360 | Fat: 0.8g | Carbs: 4.3g | Protein: 18.1g | Fiber: 0.8g | Sugar: 0g

150) **Best Paleo Beef Stew**

It's a delightful stew! The meat is so tender and succulent! It's divine!

Preparation Time: 30 minutes   **Servings: 4**

Ingredients:

- ✓ 2 lb. beef fillet, cubed
- ✓ 1 red chili, seeded and chopped
- ✓ 1 brown onion, finely chopped
- ✓ 1 tsp. ghee
- ✓ 2 tbsp. extra virgin olive oil
- ✓ Salt and black pepper to taste
- ✓ ⅔ tsp. nutmeg
- ✓ 2 tbsp. Worcestershire sauce, gluten free
- ✓ 1 garlic clove, minced
- ✓ ½ cup dried mushrooms
- ✓ ½ cup white wine
- ✓ ½ tbsp. dry sherry

Directions:

- ❖ Heat up a pot with the ghee and the olive oil over medium-high heat, add onion, chili, some salt, and pepper, stir and cook for 2-3 minutes.
- ❖ Add meat, stir and brown it for 5 minutes.
- ❖ Add Worcestershire sauce, wine, sherry, dried mushrooms, garlic, stock, thyme, fennel, rosemary, nutmeg, and star anise, stir, bring to a boil, cover, reduce heat to low and cook for 1 hour and 10 minutes.

Ingredients:

- ✓ 1 tsp. rosemary, dry
- ✓ 4 thyme springs
- ✓ ¼ tsp. fennel seeds
- ✓ 1 star anise
- ✓ 2 celery stick, chopped
- ✓ 2 carrots, thinly sliced
- ✓ 1 quart beef stock
- ✓ 6 button mushrooms, chopped
- ✓ 2 tbsp. arrowroot flour
- ✓ 1 sweet potato, chopped
- ✓ 1 tbsp. butter

- ❖ Add celery, carrots, fresh mushrooms, potato, stir, cover and cook for 15 min.
- ❖ Increase heat to medium, uncover the pot and cook the stew for 15 min.
- ❖ In a bowl, mix arrowroot flour with a cup of liquid from the stew, stir well and pour over stew.
- ❖ Also, add butter, stir well and cook for 15 more minutes.
- ❖ Transfer to bowls and serve hot.
- ❖ Enjoy!

Nutrition: Calories 113 | Fat: 8g | Carbs: 21g | Protein: 38g | Fiber: 3g | Sugar: 7g

151) Delicious Paleo Slow Cooker Stew

Preparation Time: 2 hours

Servings:

Ingredients:
- ✓ 2 lb. beef stew meat, cubed
- ✓ 3 cups dark beer
- ✓ 7 garlic cloves, finely minced
- ✓ Salt and black pepper to taste
- ✓ 4 carrots, chopped
- ✓ 1 cup tapioca flour

Ingredients:
- ✓ 2 yellow onions, finely chopped
- ✓ ½ head cabbage, finely chopped
- ✓ 30 oz. canned tomatoes, diced
- ✓ 5 yellow potatoes, chopped
- ✓ 2 cups reserved beef marinade
- ✓ 3 cups beef stock
- ❖ Transfer meat to your slow cooker.
- ❖ Add reserved marinade, carrots, cabbage, onions, tomatoes, four garlic cloves, potatoes, beef stock, salt and pepper to the taste, cover pan and cook stew on Low for 8 hours.
- ❖ Uncover pot, transfer stew to bowls and serve.
- ❖ Enjoy!

Directions:
- ❖ In a bowl, mix beef with beer and three garlic cloves, toss to coat and keep in the fridge for one day.
- ❖ In a bowl, combine tapioca flour with salt and pepper to the taste and stir.
- ❖ Drain meat and reserve the 2 cups of the marinade.
- ❖ Add meat to tapioca bowls and toss to coat.
- ❖ Heat up a pan over medium-high heat, add chicken, stir and brown it for 2-3 minutes.

Nutrition: Calories 247 | Fat: 4.5g | Carbs: 25g | Protein: 24.2g | Fiber: 4.2g | Sugar: 1g

152) Super Paleo Veggie and Chorizo Stew

Preparation Time: 30 minutes

Servings: 4

Ingredients:
- ✓ 1 yellow onion, chopped
- ✓ 1 tbsp. coconut oil
- ✓ 2 chorizo sausages, skinless and thinly sliced
- ✓ 1 red bell pepper, chopped
- ✓ 1 carrot, thinly sliced
- ✓ 2 white potatoes, chopped
- ✓ 1 celery stick, chopped

Ingredients:
- ✓ 1 tomato, chopped
- ✓ 2 garlic cloves, finely minced
- ✓ 2 cups chicken broth
- ✓ 1 tbsp. lemon juice
- ✓ Salt and black pepper to taste
- ✓ 1 zucchini, cut
- ✓ A handful parsley leaves, finely chopped
- ❖ Add zucchini, stir, cover again and cook for ten more minutes.
- ❖ Uncover pan, cook the stew for 2 minutes more stirring often.
- ❖ Add parsley, stir, take off heat, transfer to dishes and serve.
- ❖ Enjoy!

Directions:
- ❖ Heat up a pan with the oil over medium-high heat, add chorizo, onion, celery and carrot, stir and cook for 3 minutes.
- ❖ Add red bell pepper, tomatoes, garlic, and potato, stir and cook 1 minute.
- ❖ Add lemon juice, stock, salt, and pepper, stir, bring to a boil, cover pan, reduce heat to medium and cook for 10 minutes.

Nutrition: Calories 420 | Fat: 12g | Carbs: 45g | Protein: 33.2g | Fiber: 11g | Sugar: 0g

153) Delicious Beef and Plantain Stew

Preparation Time: 1 hour   **Servings: 4**

Ingredients:

- ✓ 6 plantains, skinless and cubed
- ✓ 2 lb. beef meat, cubed
- ✓ 3 cups collard greens, chopped
- ✓ Salt and black pepper to taste
- ✓ 3 cups water

Directions:

- ❖ In your slow cooker, mix beef with plantains, collard greens, water, paprika, garlic powder, allspice, chili powder, cayenne, salt and pepper to the taste.
- ❖ Stir, cover pot and cook on High for 5 hours.

Ingredients:

- ✓ ½ cup sweet paprika
- ✓ 3 tbsp. allspice
- ✓ ¼ cup garlic powder
- ✓ 1 tsp. chili powder
- ✓ 1 tsp. cayenne pepper
- ❖ Uncover slow cooker, leave stew to cool down for a few minutes, transfer to bowls and serve.
- ❖ Enjoy!

Nutrition: Calories 410 | Fat: 11g | Carbs: 39g | Protein: 34g | Fiber: 10g | Sugar: 0g

154) Healthy Paleo Chicken Stew

Preparation Time: 2 hours   **Servings: 6**

Ingredients:

- ✓ 5 garlic cloves, finely chopped
- ✓ 2 celery stalks, chopped
- ✓ 2 yellow onions, chopped
- ✓ 2 carrots, chopped
- ✓ 2 potatoes, cubed
- ✓ 30 oz. canned pumpkin puree

Directions:

- ❖ In your slow cooker, mix chicken meat with onions, carrots, celery, potatoes, garlic, pumpkin puree, chicken stock, salt, pepper, tapioca flour and cayenne, stir well, cover and cook on low for 7 hours and 50 minutes.
- ❖ Uncover slow cooker, add spinach, cover again and cook for ten more minutes.

Ingredients:

- ✓ 2 quarts chicken stock
- ✓ 2 cups chicken meat, chopped
- ✓ ¼ cup tapioca flour
- ✓ Salt and black pepper to taste
- ✓ ½ lb. baby spinach
- ✓ ¼ tsp. cayenne pepper
- ❖ Transfer to bowls and serve hot.
- ❖ Enjoy!

Nutrition: Calories 244 | Fat: 2g | Carbs: 38g | Protein: 20g | Fiber: 6g | Sugar: 0g

155) **Special White Wine Salmon Shirataki Fettucine**

Preparation Time: approx. 35 minutes

Servings: 4

Ingredients:

- ✓ 2 (8 oz) packs shirataki fettuccine
- ✓ 5 tbsp butter
- ✓ 4 salmon fillets, cubed
- ✓ Salt and black pepper to taste
- ✓ 3 garlic cloves, minced

Ingredients:

- ✓ 1 ¼ cups heavy cream
- ✓ ½ cup dry white wine
- ✓ 1 tsp lemon zest
- ✓ 1 cup baby spinach

Directions:

- ❖ Boil 2 cups of water in a pot. Strain the shirataki pasta t and rinse well under hot running water. Allow proper draining and pour the shirataki pasta into the boiling water. Cook for 3 minutes and strain again. Place a dry skillet and stir-fry the shirataki pasta until visibly dry, 1-2 minutes; set aside. Melt half of the butter in a skillet over medium heat; season the salmon with salt and pepper and cook for 8 minutes; set aside.

- ❖ Melt remaining butter to the skillet and stir in garlic. Cook for 30 seconds. Mix in heavy cream, white wine, lemon zest, salt, and pepper. Cook over low heat for 5 minutes. Stir in spinach, let wilt for 2 minutes and stir in shirataki fettuccine and salmon. Serve.

Nutrition: Calories 795; Net Carbs 9g; Fats 46g; Protein 72g

156) **Easy Saucy Salmon with Tarragon**

Preparation Time: approx. 20 minutes

Servings: 2

Ingredients:

- ✓ 2 salmon fillets
- ✓ 1 tbsp duck fat
- ✓ Salt and black pepper to taste

Ingredients:

- ✓ 2 tbsp butter
- ✓ ½ tsp tarragon, chopped
- ✓ ¼ cup heavy cream
- ❖ Cook for 30 seconds to infuse the flavors. Whisk in heavy cream and cook for 1 minute. Serve salmon topped with the sauce.

Directions:

- ❖ Season the salmon with salt and pepper. Melt the duck fat in a pan over medium heat. Add salmon and cook for 4 minutes on both sides; set aside. In the same pan, melt the butter and add the tarragon.

Nutrition: Calories 468; Net Carbs 1.5g; Fat 40g; Protein 22g

157) **Best Cheesy Baked Trout with Zucchini**

Preparation Time: approx. 40 minutes

Servings: 4

Ingredients:

- ✓ 4 deboned trout fillets
- ✓ 2 zucchinis, sliced
- ✓ 1 tbsp butter, melted

Ingredients:

- ✓ 1 cup Greek yogurt
- ✓ ¼ cup cheddar cheese, grated
- ✓ Grated Parmesan for topping
- ❖ Pour and smear the mixture on the fish and sprinkle with Parmesan cheese. Bake for 30 minutes until golden brown

Directions:

- ❖ Preheat oven to 390 F. Brush the fish and zucchini slices with melted butter. Spread them in a greased baking dish. Mix the Greek yogurt with cheddar cheese in a bowl.

Nutrition: Calories 362; Net Carbs 5.8g; Fat 23g; Protein 25g

158)   Best .Traditional Salmon Panzanella

Preparation Time: approx. 25 minutes

Ingredients:

- ✓ 1 lb skinned salmon, cut into 4 steaks each
- ✓ 8 black olives, pitted and chopped
- ✓ 1 cucumber, cubed
- ✓ Salt and black pepper to taste
- ✓ 1 tbsp capers, rinsed

Directions:

- ❖ Preheat grill to high. In a bowl, mix cucumber, black olives, salt, pepper, capers, tomatoes, white wine vinegar, onions, olive oil, and bread cubes. Let sit so the flavors to incorporate.

Nutrition: Calories 338; Net Carbs 3.1g; Fat 21g; Protein 28g

Servings: 4

Ingredients:

- ✓ 2 large tomatoes, diced
- ✓ 3 tbsp white wine vinegar
- ✓ ¼ cup thinly sliced red onions
- ✓ 3 tbsp olive oil
- ✓ 2 slices zero carb bread, cubed

- ❖ Season the salmon with salt and pepper and grill it on both sides for 8 minutes. Serve the salmon steaks warm on a bed of the salad.

159)   Special Teriyaki Salmon with Steamed Broccoli

Preparation Time:approx. 30 min + chilling time

Ingredients:

- ✓ ¼ cup grated Pecorino Romano cheese + some more
- ✓ 4 salmon fillets
- ✓ ½ cup teriyaki sauce

Directions:

- ❖ Cover the salmon with the teriyaki sauce and refrigerate for 30 minutes. Steam the broccoli rabe for 4-5 minutes until tender. Season with salt and pepper and set aside.

Nutrition: Calories 354; Net Carbs 4g; Fat 17g; Protein 28g

Servings: 4

Ingredients:

- ✓ 1 bunch of broccoli rabe
- ✓ Salt and black pepper to taste

- ❖ Preheat oven to 400 F. Remove the salmon from the fridge and place in a greased baking dish. Bake in the oven for 14-16 minutes. Serve with steamed broccoli rabe.

160)   Easy Baked Salmon with Pistachio Crust

Preparation Time: approx. 35 minutes

Ingredients:

- ✓ 4 salmon fillets
- ✓ ¼ cup mayonnaise
- ✓ ½ cup ground pistachios
- ✓ 1 chopped shallot
- ✓ 2 tsp lemon zest

Directions:

- ❖ Preheat oven to 375 F. Spread mayonnaise on the fillets. Coat with ground pistachios. Place in a lined baking dish and bake for 15 minutes. Heat the olive oil in a saucepan and sauté shallot for 3 minutes

Nutrition: Calories 563; Net Carbs 6g; Fat 47g; Protein 34g

Servings: 4

Ingredients:

- ✓ 1 tbsp olive oil
- ✓ A pinch of pepper
- ✓ 1 cup heavy cream

- ❖ Stir in heavy cream and lemon zest. Bring to a boil and cook until thickened. Pour the sauce over the salmon and serve.

161) Rich Party Smoked Salmon Balls

Preparation Time: approx 30 minutes

Servings: 6

Ingredients:
- 12 oz sliced smoked salmon, finely chopped
- 1 parsnip, cooked and mashed
- Salt and chili pepper to taste
- 4 tbsp olive oil

Directions:
- In a bowl, add the salmon, eggs, pesto sauce, pork rinds, salt, and chili pepper. Mix well and make 6 compact balls.

Ingredients:
- 2 eggs, beaten
- 2 tbsp pesto sauce
- 1 tbsp pork rinds, crushed

- Heat olive oil in a skillet over medium heat and fry the balls for 3 minutes on each side until golden brown. Remove to a wire rack to cool. Serve warm.

Nutrition: Calories 254; Net Carbs 4.3g; Fat 18g; Protein 17g

162) Italian Salmon Caesar Salad with Poached Eggs

Preparation Time: approx. 15 minutes

Servings: 4

Ingredients:
- ½ cup chopped smoked salmon
- 2 tbsp heinz low carb caesar dressing
- 3 cups water

Directions:
- Boil water in a pot over medium heat. Crack each egg into a small bowl and gently slide into the water. Poach for 2-3 minutes, remove, and transfer to a plate.

Ingredients:
- 8 eggs
- 2 cups torn romaine lettuce
- 4 pancetta slices
- Poach the remaining eggs. Put the pancetta in a skillet and fry for 6 minutes, turning once. Allow cooling and chop into small pieces. Toss the lettuce, smoked salmon, pancetta, and caesar dressing in a salad bowl. Top with the eggs.

Nutrition: Calories 260; Net Carbs 5g; Fat 21g; Protein 8g

163) Special Mahi Mahi with Dill Sour Cream Topping

Preparation Time: approx. 30 minutes

Servings: 4

Ingredients:
- ½ cup grated Pecorino Romano cheese
- 1 cup sour cream
- ½ tbsp minced dill

Directions:
- Preheat oven to 400 F. Line a baking sheet with parchment paper. In a bowl, mix sour cream, dill, and lemon zest; set aside. Drizzle the mahi mahi with lemon juice and arrange on the baking sheet.

Ingredients:
- ½ lemon, zested and juiced
- 4 mahi mahi fillets

- Spread sour cream mixture on top and sprinkle with Pecorino Romano cheese. Bake for 15 minutes. Broil the top for 2 minutes until nicely brown. Serve with buttery green beans.

Nutrition: Calories 288; Net Carbs 1.2g; Fat 23g; Protein 16g

164) **Paleo Mediterranean Tilapia**

Preparation Time: approx. 30 minutes

Servings: 4

Ingredients:

- ✓ 4 tilapia fillets
- ✓ 2 garlic cloves, minced
- ✓ ½ tsp dry oregano
- ✓ 14 oz canned diced tomatoes

Ingredients:

- ✓ 2 tbsp olive oil
- ✓ ½ red onion, chopped
- ✓ 1 tbsp fresh parsley, chopped
- ✓ ¼ cup kalamata olives
- ❖ Add olives and tilapia. Cook for 8 minutes. Serve topped with parsley.

Directions:

- ❖ Heat oil in a skillet over medium heat and cook onion for 3 minutes. Add garlic and oregano and cook for 30 seconds.
- ❖ Stir in tomatoes and bring the mixture to a boil. Reduce the heat and simmer for 5 minutes.

Nutrition: Calories 182; Net Carbs 6g; Fat 15g; Protein 23g

165) **Easy Paleo Lamb and Coconut Stew**

Preparation Time: 1 hour 15 minutes

Servings: 4

Ingredients:

- ✓ 1 and ½ lb. lamb meat, diced
- ✓ 1 tbsp. coconut oil
- ✓ ½ red chili, seedless and chopped
- ✓ 1 brown onion, chopped
- ✓ 3 garlic cloves, minced
- ✓ 2 celery sticks, chopped
- ✓ 2 and ½ tsp. garam masala powder
- ✓ 1 tsp. fennel seeds
- ✓ Salt and black pepper to taste

Ingredients:

- ✓ 1 and ¼ tsp. turmeric
- ✓ 1 and ½ tsp. ghee
- ✓ 14 oz. canned coconut milk
- ✓ 1 and ½ tbsp. coconut milk
- ✓ 1 cup water
- ✓ 1 tbsp. lemon juice
- ✓ 2 carrots, chopped
- ✓ A handful parsley leaves, finely chopped

- ❖ Add salt, pepper to the taste, tomato paste, coconut milk, and water, stir, bring to a boil, reduce heat to low, cover and cook for 1 hour.
- ❖ Add carrots and cook fro 40 minutes more, stirring from time to time.
- ❖ Add lemon juice and parsley, stir, take off heat, transfer to bowls and serve.
- ❖ Enjoy!

Directions:

- ❖ Heat up a pan with the oil over medium-high heat, add lamb, stir and brown for 4 minutes.
- ❖ Add celery, chili and onion, stir and cook 1 minute.
- ❖ Reduce heat to medium, add garam masala, garlic, ghee, fennel, and turmeric, stir and cook 1 minute.

Nutrition: Calories 450 | Fat: 31g | Carbs: 40g | Protein: 50g | Fiber: 1g | Sugar: 0g

166) Special Paleo Veggie Stew

Preparation Time: 30 minutes   **Servings: 4**

Ingredients:

- ✓ 4 lb. mixed root vegetables (parsnips, carrots, rutabagas, potatoes, beets, celery root, turnips), chopped
- ✓ 6 tbsp. extra virgin olive oil
- ✓ 1 garlic head, cloves separated and peeled
- ✓ ½ cup yellow onion, chopped
- ✓ Salt and black pepper to taste

Directions:

- ❖ In a baking dish, mix all root vegetables with salt, pepper, half of the oil and garlic, toss to coat, introduce in the oven at 450 degrees G and roast them for 45 minutes.
- ❖ Heat up a pot with the rest of the oil over medium-high heat, add onions and cook for 2-3 minutes stirring often.
- ❖ Add tomato paste, stir and cook one more minute.

Ingredients:

- ✓ 28 oz. canned tomatoes, peeled and chopped
- ✓ 1 tbsp. tomato paste
- ✓ 2 cups kale leaves, torn
- ✓ 1 tsp. oregano, dried
- ✓ Tabasco sauce for serving

- ❖ Add tomatoes and their liquid, some salt and pepper and the oregano, stir, bring to a simmer, reduce heat to low and cook until veggies become roasted.
- ❖ Take root vegetables out of the oven, add them to the pot and stir.
- ❖ Add kale, stir and cook for 5 minutes.
- ❖ Add Tabasco sauce to the taste, mix, transfer to bowls and serve.
- ❖ Enjoy!

Nutrition: Calories 150 | Fat: 7g | Carbs: 17.2g | Protein: 2.4g | Fiber: 3.7g | Sugar: 0g

167) Easy Paleo French Chicken Stew

Preparation Time: 30 minutes   **Servings: 4**

Ingredients:

- ✓ 10 garlic cloves, peeled
- ✓ 30 black olives, pitted
- ✓ 2 lb. chicken pieces
- ✓ 2 cups chicken stock
- ✓ 28 oz. canned tomatoes, chopped

Directions:

- ❖ Heat up a pot with some olive oil over medium-high heat, add chicken pieces, salt, and pepper to the taste and cook for 4 minutes, stirring often.
- ❖ Add garlic, stir and brown for 2 minutes.
- ❖ Add chicken stock, tomatoes, olives, thyme, and rosemary, stir, cover pot and bake in the oven at 325 degrees for 1 hour.

Ingredients:

- ✓ 2 tbsp. rosemary, chopped
- ✓ 2 tbsp. parsley leaves, chopped
- ✓ 2 tbsp. basil leaves, chopped
- ✓ Salt and black pepper to taste
- ✓ A drizzle of extra virgin olive oil
- ❖ Add parsley and basil, mix, introduce in the oven again and bake for 45 more minutes.
- ❖ Leave stew to cool down for a few minutes, transfer to plates and serve.
- ❖ Enjoy!

Nutrition: Calories 300 | Fat: 48g | Carbs: 16g | Protein: 61g | Fiber: 6g | Sugar: 0g

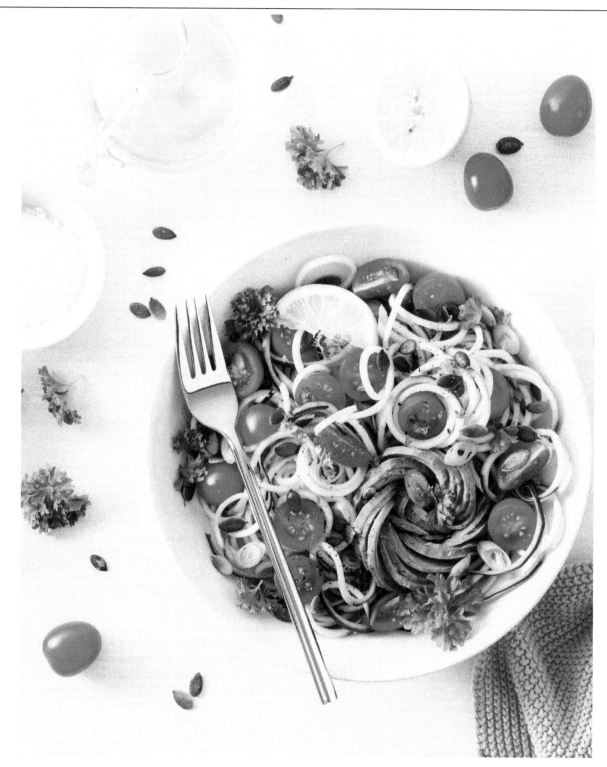

168) **Mint ice cream**

Preparation Time: 10 minutes + cooling time

Servings: 4

Ingredients:
- ✓ 2 avocados, pitted
- ✓ 1 ¼ cup coconut cream
- ✓ ½ tsp vanilla extract

Ingredients:
- ✓ 2 tbsp erythritol
- ✓ 2 tbsp chopped mint leaves

Directions:
- ❖ In a blender, pour the avocado pulp, coconut cream, vanilla extract, erythritol and mint leaves. Process until the mixture is smooth.

- ❖ Pour the mixture into the ice cream maker and freeze according to the manufacturer's instructions. When ready, remove and pour ice cream into a bowl.

Nutrition: Calories 370; Net carbohydrates 4g; Fat 38g; Protein 4g

169) **Pizza with sweet onion and goat cheese**

Preparation Time: 35 minutes

Servings: 4

Ingredients:
- ✓ 2 cups grated mozzarella cheese
- ✓ 2 tbsp cream cheese, softened
- ✓ 2 large eggs, beaten
- ✓ ⅓ cup almond flour
- ✓ 1 tsp dry Italian seasoning

Ingredients:
- ✓ 2 tbsp butter
- ✓ 2 red onions, thinly sliced
- ✓ 1 cup crumbled goat cheese
- ✓ 1 tbsp almond milk
- ✓ 1 cup curly endive, chopped

Directions:
- ❖ Preheat oven to 390 F. Line a round pizza pan with baking paper. Microwave the mozzarella and cream cheeses for 1 minute. Remove and mix in the eggs, almond flour and Italian seasoning. Spread the mixture on the baking sheet and bake for 6 minutes.

- ❖ Melt butter in a skillet and stir in onions, salt and pepper and cook over low heat and stirring often until caramelized, 15-20 minutes. In a bowl, mix the goat cheese with the almond milk and spread over the crust. Top with the caramelized onions. Bake for 10 minutes. Scatter curly endive over the top, slice and serve.

Nutrition: Calories 317; Net Carbs 3g; Fat 20g; Protein 28g

170) **Pizza with spinach and olives**

Preparation Time: 40 minutes

Servings: 4

Ingredients:
- ✓ 1 cup grated mozzarella cheese
- ✓ ½ cup almond flour
- ✓ ¼ tsp salt
- ✓ 2 tbsp ground psyllium husk
- ✓ 1 tbsp olive oil

Ingredients:
- ✓ 1 cup warm water
- ✓ ½ cup of tomato sauce
- ✓ ½ cup baby spinach
- ✓ 1 tsp dried oregano
- ✓ 3 tbsp sliced black olives

Directions:
- ❖ Preheat oven to 390 F. Line a baking sheet with parchment paper. In a bowl, mix the almond flour, salt, psyllium husk, olive oil and water until a dough forms. Spread the dough on the sheet and bake for 10 minutes

- ❖ Remove the crust and spread the tomato sauce on top. Add the spinach, mozzarella, oregano and olives. Bake for 15 minutes. Remove from oven, slice and serve warm.

Nutrition: Calories 195; Net Carbs 1.8g; Fat 8g; Protein 11g

171) Tofu Nuggets with cilantro sauce

Preparation Time: 25 minutes

Servings: 4

Ingredients:

- ✓ 1 lime, ½ squeezed and ½ cut into wedges
- ✓ 1 ½ cups olive oil
- ✓ 28 ounces tofu, pressed and diced
- ✓ 1 egg, lightly beaten
- ✓ 1 cup golden flax seed meal

Directions:

- ❖ Heat the olive oil in a deep skillet. Coat the tofu cubes in the egg and then in the flaxseed meal. Fry until golden brown.

Ingredients:

- ✓ 1 ripe avocado, chopped
- ✓ ½ tbsp chopped cilantro
- ✓ Salt and black pepper to taste
- ✓ ½ tbsp olive oil

- ❖ Transfer to a plate. Place the avocado, cilantro, salt, pepper and lime juice in a blender; blend until smooth. Pour into a bowl, add the tofu nuggets and lime wedges to serve.

Nutrition: Calories 665; Net carbs 6.2g, fat 54g, protein 32g

172) Spicy Brussels sprouts with carrots

Preparation Time: 15 minutes

Servings: 4

Ingredients:

- ✓ 1 pound Brussels sprouts
- ✓ ¼ cup olive oil
- ✓ 4 green onions, chopped

Directions:

- ❖ Sauté green onions in hot olive oil for 2 minutes. Sprinkle with salt and pepper and transfer to a plate. Cut the Brussels sprouts and split them in half.

Ingredients:

- ✓ 2 carrots, grated
- ✓ Salt and black pepper to taste
- ✓ Hot chili sauce
- ❖ Leave the small ones as whole. Pour the Brussels sprouts and carrots into the same saucepan and sauté until softened but al dente. Season to taste and toss with the onions. Cook for 3 minutes. Add chili sauce and serve.

Nutrition: Calories 198; Net carbohydrates 6.5g; Fat 14g; Protein 4.9g

173) Zucchini-Cranberry Cake Squares

Preparation Time: 45 minutes

Servings: 6

Ingredients:

- ✓ 1 ¼ cups chopped zucchini
- ✓ 2 tbsp olive oil
- ✓ ½ cup dried cranberries
- ✓ 1 lemon, peeled
- ✓ 3 eggs

Directions:

- ❖ Preheat oven to 350 F. Line a square cake pan with baking paper. Combine the zucchini, olive oil, cranberries, lemon zest and eggs in a bowl until evenly combined.

Ingredients:

- ✓ 1 ½ cups almond flour
- ✓ ½ tsp baking powder
- ✓ 1 tsp cinnamon powder
- ✓ A pinch of salt

- ❖ Add the almond flour, baking powder, cinnamon powder and salt into the mixture. Pour the mixture into the cake pan and bake for 30 minutes. Remove from the oven, let cool in the cake pan for 10 minutes and transfer the cake to a wire rack to cool completely. Cut into squares and serve.

Nutrition: Calories 121; Net Carbs 2.5g, Fat 10g, Protein 4g

174) Fried rice egg with grilled cheese

Preparation Time: 10 minutes

Servings: 4

Ingredients:

- ✓ 2 cups cauliflower rice, steamed
- ✓ ½ pound halloumi, cut into ¼- to ½-inch slabs
- ✓ 1 tbsp ghee
- ✓ 4 eggs, beaten

Directions:

- ❖ Melt the ghee in a skillet and pour in the eggs. Rotate the pan to scatter the eggs and cook for 1 minute. Move the scrambled eggs to the side of the skillet, add the bell bell pepper and green beans and saute for 3 minutes. Pour in the cauli rice and cook for 2 minutes.

Ingredients:

- ✓ 1 green bell pepper, chopped
- ✓ ¼ cup green beans, chopped
- ✓ 1 tsp soy sauce
- ✓ 2 tbsp chopped parsley
- ❖ Add the soy sauce; combine evenly and cook for 2 minutes. Distribute to plates, garnish with parsley and set aside. Preheat a grill pan and grill halloumi cheese on both sides until cheese turns slightly brown. Place on the side of the rice and serve hot.

Nutrition: Calories 275; Net carbs 4.5g, fat 19g, protein 15g

175) Fake Mushroom Risotto

Preparation Time: 15 minutes

Servings: 4

Ingredients:

- ✓ 2 shallots, diced
- ✓ 3 tbsp olive oil
- ✓ ¼ cup vegetable stock
- ✓ ⅓ cup Parmesan cheese

Directions:

- ❖ Heat 2 tbsp oil in a saucepan, add mushrooms and cook over medium heat for 3 minutes.

Ingredients:

- ✓ 4 tbsp butter
- ✓ 3 tbsp chopped chives
- ✓ 2 pounds mushrooms, sliced
- ✓ 4 1/2 cups rinsed cauliflower
- ❖ Remove and set aside. Heat the remaining oil and cook the shallots for 2 minutes. Add the cauliflower and broth and cook until the liquid is absorbed. Stir in the rest of the ingredients.

Nutrition: Calories 264; Net carbs 8.4g; Fat 18g; Protein 11g

176) Eggplant pizza with cheese

Preparation Time: 40 minutes

Servings: 2

Ingredients:

- ✓ 6 ounces grated mozzarella cheese
- ✓ 2 tbsp cream cheese
- ✓ 2 tbsp Parmesan cheese
- ✓ 1 tsp oregano
- ✓ ½ cup almond flour
- ✓ 2 tbsp psyllium husk

Directions:

- ❖ Preheat oven to 400 F. Melt the mozzarella cheese in the microwave. Combine cream cheese, Parmesan cheese, oregano, almond flour and psyllium husk in a bowl. Add the melted mozzarella cheese and stir to combine.

Ingredients:

- ✓ 4 ounces grated cheddar cheese
- ✓ ¼ cup marinara sauce
- ✓ Eggplant, sliced
- ✓ 1 tomato, sliced
- ✓ 2 tbsp chopped basil
- ✓ 6 black olives
- ❖ Divide the dough into 2. Roll out the crusts into circles and place on a lined baking sheet. Bake for 10 minutes. Add the cheddar cheese, marinara, eggplant, tomato and basil. Return to oven and bake for 10 minutes. Serve with olives.

Nutrition: Calories 510; Net Carbs 3.7g; Fat 39g; Protein 31g

177)   Eggplant and Goat Cheese Pizza

Preparation Time: 45   minutes

Servings: 4

Ingredients:
- ✓ 4 tbsp olive oil
- ✓ 2 eggplants, sliced lengthwise
- ✓ 1 cup tomato sauce
- ✓ 2 garlic cloves, minced
- ✓ 1 red onion, sliced
- ✓ 12 ounces goat cheese, crumbled

Ingredients:
- ✓ Salt and black pepper to taste
- ✓ ½ tsp cinnamon powder
- ✓ 1 cup mozzarella cheese, shredded
- ✓ 2 tbsp oregano, chopped

Directions:
- ❖ Line a baking sheet with baking paper. Arrange eggplant slices on baking sheet and drizzle with a little olive oil. Bake for 20 minutes at 390 F. Heat the remaining olive oil in a skillet and sauté the garlic and onion for 3 minutes.

- ❖ Add goat cheese and tomato sauce and season with salt and pepper. Simmer for 10 minutes. Remove eggplant from oven and spread cheese sauce on top. Sprinkle with mozzarella cheese and oregano. Bake for 10 minutes more until cheese melts. Cut into slices and serve.

Nutrition: Calories 557; Net Carbs 8.3g; Fat 44g; Protein 33g

178)   Mushroom and broccoli pizza

Preparation Time: 25   minutes

Servings: 4

Ingredients:
- ✓ ½ cup almond flour
- ✓ ¼ tsp salt
- ✓ 2 tbsp ground psyllium husk
- ✓ 2 tbsp olive oil
- ✓ 1 cup fresh sliced mushrooms
- ✓ 1 white onion, thinly sliced

Ingredients:
- ✓ 3 cups broccoli florets
- ✓ 2 cloves garlic, minced
- ✓ ½ cup unsweetened pizza sauce
- ✓ 4 tomatoes, sliced
- ✓ 1 ½ cups mozzarella cheese, grated
- ✓ ⅓ cup grated Parmesan cheese

Directions:
- ❖ Preheat oven to 390 F. Line a baking sheet with parchment paper. In a bowl, mix almond flour, salt, psyllium powder, 1 tbsp olive oil and 1 cup warm water until a dough forms. Spread the dough onto the pizza pan and bake for 10 minutes.

- ❖ Heat the remaining olive oil in a skillet and sauté mushrooms, onion, garlic and broccoli for 5 minutes. Spread the pizza sauce over the crust and top with the broccoli mixture, tomato, mozzarella and Parmesan. Bake for 5 minutes. Serve in slices.

Nutrition: Calories 180; Net carbs 3.6g; Fat 9g; Protein 17g

179)   Tofu radish bowls

Preparation Time: 35   minutes

Servings: 4

Ingredients:
- ✓ ¼ cup baby mushrooms, chopped
- ✓ 2 yellow peppers, chopped
- ✓ 1 block of tofu (14 oz), cubed
- ✓ 1 tbsp + 1 tbsp olive oil
- ✓ 1 ½ cups shredded radishes

Ingredients:
- ✓ ½ cup chopped white onions
- ✓ 4 eggs
- ✓ 1/3 cup tomato sauce
- ✓ A handful of chopped parsley
- ✓ 1 avocado, and chopped

Directions:
- ❖ Heat 1 tbsp olive oil in a skillet and add tofu, radishes, onions, mushrooms and peppers; cook for 10 minutes. Divide among 4 bowls. Heat the remaining oil in the skillet, crack an egg into the pan

- ❖ Transfer to the top of a bowl of tofu hash and make the remaining eggs. Top the bowls with the tomato sauce, parsley and avocado. Serve.

and cook until the white sets but the yolk is quite runny.

Nutrition: Calories 353; Net Carbs 5.9g, Fat 25g, Protein 19g

180) Tomato & Mozzarella Caprese Bake

Preparation Time: 25 minutes   **Servings: 4**

Ingredients:
- ✓ 4 tbsp olive oil
- ✓ 4 tomatoes, sliced
- ✓ 1 cup fresh mozzarella, sliced

Directions:
- ❖ In a baking dish, arrange the tomatoes and mozzarella slices. In a bowl, mix the pesto, mayonnaise and half of the Parmesan cheese; stir to combine.

Ingredients:
- ✓ 2 tbsp basil pesto
- ✓ 1 cup mayonnaise
- ✓ 2 ounces Parmesan cheese, grated
- ❖ Spread this mixture over the tomatoes and mozzarella and top with the remaining Parmesan cheese. Bake for 20 minutes at 360 F. Remove, let cool slightly and slice to serve.

Nutrition: Calories 420; Net Carbs 4.9g; Fat 36g; Protein 17g

181) Cookies with heart of pistachio

Preparation Time: 30 min + cooling time   **Servings: 4**

Ingredients:
- ✓ 1 cup butter, softened
- ✓ 2/3 cup sugar swerve
- ✓ 1 large egg, beaten
- ✓ 2 tsp pistachio extract

Directions:
- ❖ Add the butter and swerve sugar to a bowl and beat until smooth and creamy. Beat in the egg until combined. Stir in the pistachio extract and almond flour until a smooth dough forms. Wrap the dough in plastic wrap and chill for 10 minutes. Preheat oven to 350 F. Lightly dust a cutting board with almond flour. Unroll the dough and roll it out to a thickness of 2 inches.

Ingredients:
- ✓ 2 cups almond flour
- ✓ ½ cup dark chocolate
- ✓ 2 tbsp chopped pistachios
- ❖ Cut out as many cookies as you can get, while rolling back the scraps to make more cookies. Place the cookies on the baking sheet lined with parchment paper and bake for 15 minutes. Transfer to a wire rack to cool completely. Melt the dark chocolate in the microwave. Dip one side of each cookie into the melted chocolate. Garnish chocolate side with pistachios and let cool on a wire rack. Serve.

Nutrition: Calories 470; Net carbs 3.4g, fat 45g, protein 6.2g

182)   **Avocado and tomato burritos**

Preparation Time: 10   minutes

Servings: 4

Ingredients:
- ✓ 2 cups cauli rice
- ✓ 6 low carb tortillas
- ✓ 2 cups sour cream sauce

Directions:
- ❖ Pour cauli rice into a bowl, sprinkle with a little water, and microwave for 2 minutes to soften. On the tortillas, spread the sour cream and spread the salsa on top.

Ingredients:
- ✓ 1 ½ cups herbed tomato sauce
- ✓ 2 avocados, peeled, pitted and sliced

- ❖ Top with the cauli rice and spread the avocado evenly on top. Fold and tuck the burritos and cut in half. Serve.

Nutrition: Calories 303, Fat 25g, Net Carbs 6g, Protein 8g

183)   **Creamy cucumber and avocado soup**

Preparation Time: 15   minutes

Servings: 4

Ingredients:
- ✓ 4 large cucumbers, seeded and cut into pieces
- ✓ 1 large avocado, peeled and cut in half
- ✓ Salt and black pepper to taste
- ✓ 1 tbsp fresh cilantro, chopped
- ✓ 3 tbsp olive oil

Directions:
- ❖ Pour cucumbers, avocado halves, salt, black pepper, olive oil, lime juice, cilantro, 2 cups water and garlic into food processor. Puree the ingredients for 2 minutes or until smooth.

Ingredients:
- ✓ 2 limes, squeezed
- ✓ 2 tbsp minced garlic
- ✓ 2 tomatoes, chopped
- ✓ 1 avocado, chopped for garnish

- ❖ Pour mixture into a bowl and top with avocado and chopped tomatoes. Serve cold with zero carb bread.

Nutrition: Calories 170, Fat 7.4g, Net Carbs 4.1g, Protein 3.7g

184)   **Cauliflower "couscous" with lemon and Halloumi**

Preparation Time: 5   minutes

Servings: 4

Ingredients:
- ✓ 4 ounces of halloumi, sliced
- ✓ 2 tbsp olive oil
- ✓ 1 head of cauliflower, cut into florets
- ✓ ¼ cup chopped cilantro

Directions:
- ❖ Heat the olive oil in a skillet over medium heat. Add halloumi and fry for 2 minutes on each side until golden brown; set aside. Pour the cauli florets into a food processor and pulse until it crumbles and resembles couscous. Transfer to a bowl and steam in the microwave for 2 minutes.

Ingredients:
- ✓ ¼ cup chopped parsley
- ✓ ¼ cup chopped mint
- ✓ ½ lemon, squeezed
- ✓ Salt and black pepper to taste
- ✓ 1 avocado, sliced for garnish

- ❖ Remove the bowl from the microwave and allow the cauli to cool. Add the cilantro, parsley, mint, lemon juice, salt and pepper. Top the couscous with avocado slices and serve with grilled halloumi and vegetable sauce.

Nutrition: Calories 185, Fat 15.6g, Net Carbs 2.1g, Protein 12g

185) **Zucchini lasagna with ricotta cheese and spinach**

Preparation Time: 50 minutes

Servings: 4

Ingredients:
- ✓ 2 zucchini, sliced
- ✓ Salt and black pepper to taste
- ✓ 2 cups ricotta cheese

Directions:
- ❖ Preheat oven to 370°F. Place zucchini slices in a colander and sprinkle with salt. Let stand and drain liquid for 5 minutes and pat dry with paper towels. Mix the ricotta, mozzarella, salt and black pepper to combine evenly and spread ¼ cup of the mixture over the bottom of the baking dish.
- ❖ Arrange ⅓ of the zucchini slices on top, spread 1 cup of the tomato sauce, and scatter ⅓ cup of the spinach on top.

Ingredients:
- ✓ 2 cups shredded mozzarella cheese
- ✓ 3 cups tomato sauce
- ✓ 1 cup spinach
- ❖ Repeat the layering process two more times to run out of ingredients, finally making sure to layer with the last ¼ cup of cheese mixture.
- ❖ Grease one end of the aluminum foil with cooking spray and cover the baking sheet with the foil. Bake for 35 minutes, remove the foil and bake further for 5-10 minutes or until the cheese has a nice golden brown color. Remove dish, let rest for 5 minutes, make lasagna slices and serve warm.

186) Briam with tomato sauce

Preparation Time: 40 minutes

Servings: 4

Ingredients:
- ✓ 3 tbsp olive oil
- ✓ 1 large eggplant, halved and sliced
- ✓ 1 large onion, thinly sliced
- ✓ 3 garlic cloves, sliced
- ✓ 2 tomatoes, diced
- ✓ 1 rutabaga, diced

Directions:
- ❖ Preheat oven to 400°F. Heat the olive oil in a skillet over medium heat and fry the eggplant and zucchini slices for 6 minutes until golden brown. Remove them to a casserole dish and arrange them in a single layer.

Ingredients:
- ✓ 1 cup unsweetened tomato sauce
- ✓ 4 zucchini, sliced
- ✓ ¼ cup water
- ✓ Salt and black pepper to taste
- ✓ ¼ tsp dried oregano
- ✓ 2 tbsp fresh parsley, chopped
- ❖ Sauté the onion and garlic in the oil for 3 minutes. Remove to a bowl. Add the tomatoes, rutabaga, tomato sauce and water and mix well. Stir in salt, pepper, oregano and parsley. Pour the mixture over the eggplant and zucchini. Place the dish in the oven and bake for 25-30 minutes. Serve the briam hot.

Nutrition: Calories Calories 365, Fat 12g, Net Carbohydrates 12.5g, Protein 11.3g

187) **Creamy vegetable stew**

Preparation Time: 25 minutes

Servings: 4

Ingredients:
- ✓ 2 tbsp ghee
- ✓ 1 tbsp onion and garlic puree
- ✓ 2 medium carrots, shredded
- ✓ 1 head of cauliflower, cut into florets

Directions:
- ❖ Melt ghee in a saucepan over medium heat and sauté onion and garlic puree to be fragrant, 2 minutes. Stir

Ingredients:
- ✓ 2 cups green beans, cut in half
- ✓ Salt and black pepper to taste
- ✓ 1 cup water
- ✓ 1 ½ cups heavy cream
- ❖ Pour in water, stir again and cook over low heat for 15 minutes. Stir in the heavy cream to incorporate and turn off the heat. Serve the stew with almond flour bread.

in carrots, cauliflower and green beans for 5 minutes. Season with salt and black pepper.

Nutrition: Calories 310, fat 26.4g, net carbs 6g, protein 8g

188)   Tempeh kabobs with vegetables

Preparation Time: 30 minutes + cooling time

Servings: 4

Ingredients:

✓   2 tbsp ghee
✓   1 tbsp onion and garlic puree
✓   2 medium carrots, shredded
✓   1 head of cauliflower, cut into florets

Directions:

❖   Melt ghee in a saucepan over medium heat and sauté onion and garlic puree to be fragrant, 2 minutes. Stir in carrots, cauliflower and green beans for 5 minutes. Season with salt and black pepper.

Ingredients:

✓   2 cups green beans, cut in half
✓   Salt and black pepper to taste
✓   1 cup water
✓   1 ½ cups heavy cream
❖   Pour in water, stir again and cook over low heat for 15 minutes. Stir in the heavy cream to incorporate and turn off the heat. Serve the stew with almond flour bread.

Nutrition: Calories Calories 228, Fat 15g, Net Carbohydrates 3.6g, Protein 13.2g

189)   Tempeh kabobs with vegetables

Preparation Time: 30 minutes + cooling time

Servings: 4

Ingredients:

✓   1 yellow bell pepper, cut into pieces
✓   10 ounces tempeh, cut into pieces
✓   1 red onion, cut into pieces

Directions:

❖   Bring the 1 ½ cups of water to a boil in a pot over medium heat, and once it's cooked, turn off the heat and add the tempeh. Cover the pot and allow the tempeh to steam for 5 minutes to remove the bitterness. Drain. Pour barbecue sauce into a bowl, add tempeh and coat with sauce. Refrigerate for 2 hours.

Ingredients:

✓   1 red bell bell pepper, cut into pieces
✓   2 tbsp olive oil
✓   1 cup unsweetened barbecue sauce
❖   Preheat grill to 350°F. Thread the tempeh, yellow bell pepper, red bell pepper and onion onto skewers. Brush the grill grate with olive oil, place the skewers on and brush with the barbecue sauce. Cook skewers for 3 minutes on each side, rotating and brushing with more barbecue sauce. Serve.

Nutrition: Calories Calories 228, Fat 15g, Net Carbohydrates 3.6g, Protein 13.2g

190)   Cauliflower and Gouda Cheese Casserole

Preparation Time: 25 minutes

Servings: 4

Ingredients:

✓   2 heads of cauliflower, cut into florets
✓   2 tbsp olive oil
✓   2 tbsp melted butter
✓   1 white onion, chopped

Directions:

❖   Preheat oven to 350°F. Place cauli florets in a large microwave-safe bowl. Sprinkle with a little water and steam in the microwave for 4 to 5 minutes. Heat the olive oil in a saucepan over medium heat and sauté

Ingredients:

✓   Salt and black pepper to taste
✓   ¼ cup almond milk
✓   ½ cup almond flour
✓   1 ½ cups gouda cheese, grated
❖   Cook over low heat for 3 minutes. Mix the melted butter with the almond flour. Stir in the cauliflower and half of the cheese. Sprinkle the top with the remaining cheese and bake for 10 minutes until the cheese is melted and golden brown on top. Plate the oven and serve with the salad.

the onion for 3 minutes. Add the cauliflower, season with salt and pepper and stir in the almond milk.

Nutrition: Calories 215, Fat 15g, Net Carbs 4g, Protein 12g

191)   Roasted Asparagus with Spicy Eggplant Sauce

Preparation Time: 35 minutes   **Servings: 6**

Ingredients:

- ✓   1 ½ pounds asparagus, chopped
- ✓   ¼ cup + 2 tbsp olive oil
- ✓   ½ tsp paprika
- ✓   Eggplant Sauce
- ✓   1 pound of eggplant
- ✓   ½ cup shallots, chopped

Directions:

- ❖   Preheat oven to 390°F. Line a parchment paper on a baking sheet. Add the asparagus. Season with 2 tbsp olive oil, paprika, black pepper and salt. Roast until cooked through, 9 minutes. Remove.
- ❖   Place the eggplant on a cookie sheet lined baking sheet. Bake in the oven for about 20 minutes.

Ingredients:

- ✓   2 cloves garlic, minced
- ✓   1 tbsp fresh lemon juice
- ✓   ½ tsp chili pepper
- ✓   Salt and black pepper to taste
- ✓   ¼ cup fresh cilantro, chopped

- ❖   Allow eggplant to cool. Peel them and discard the stems. Heat the remaining olive oil in a skillet over medium heat and add the garlic and shallots. Sauté for 3 minutes until tender.
- ❖   In a food processor, put together the black pepper, roasted eggplant, salt, lemon juice, shallot mixture, and red pepper. Add the cilantro and serve alongside the roasted asparagus spears.

Nutrition: Calories 149; Fat: 12.1g, Net Carbohydrates: 9g, Protein: 3.6g

192)   Cook the squash

Preparation Time: 45 minutes   **Servings: 6**

Ingredients:

- ✓   3 large pumpkins, peeled and sliced
- ✓   1 cup almond flour
- ✓   1 cup grated mozzarella cheese

Directions:

- ❖   Preheat oven to 350°F. Arrange the squash slices in a baking dish and drizzle with olive oil.

Ingredients:

- ✓   3 tbsp olive oil
- ✓   ½ cup fresh parsley, chopped

- ❖   Bake for 35 minutes. Mix almond flour, mozzarella cheese and parsley and pour over squash. Return to oven and bake for another 5 minutes until top is golden brown. Serve warm.

Nutrition: Calories 125, Fat 4.8g, Net Carbs 5.7g, Protein 2.7g

193)   Cremini Mushroom Stroganoff

Preparation Time: 25 minutes   **Servings: 4**

Ingredients:

- ✓   3 tbsp butter
- ✓   1 white onion, chopped
- ✓   4 cups cremini mushrooms, diced

Directions:

- ❖   Melt the butter in a saucepan over medium heat and sauté the onion for 3 minutes until soft. Add the mushrooms and cook until tender, about 5 minutes. Add 2 cups of water and bring to a boil.

Ingredients:

- ✓   ½ cup heavy cream
- ✓   ½ cup Parmesan cheese, grated
- ✓   1 ½ tbsp dried mixed herbs
- ❖   Cook for 10-15 minutes until the water reduces slightly. Pour in the heavy cream and Parmesan cheese. Stir to dissolve the cheese. Add the dried herbs and season. Simmer for 5 minutes. Serve hot.

Nutrition: Calories 284, Fat 28g, Net Carbs 1.5g, Protein 8g

194) **Portobello Mushroom Burger**

Preparation Time: 15 minutes   **Servings: 4**

Ingredients:

- ✓ 8 large portobello mushroom caps
- ✓ 1 minced garlic clove
- ✓ ½ cup of mayonnaise
- ✓ ½ tsp salt
- ✓ 4 tbsp olive oil
- ✓ ½ cup roasted red peppers, sliced

Directions:

- ❖ Preheat a grill over medium-high heat. In a bowl, crush the garlic with the salt using the back of a spoon. Stir in half the oil and brush the mushrooms and halloumi cheese with the mixture.
- ❖ Place the "sandwiches" on the skillet and grill them on both sides for 8 minutes until tender.

Ingredients:

- ✓ 2 medium tomatoes, chopped
- ✓ 4 halloumi slices, half-inch thick
- ✓ 1 tbsp red wine vinegar
- ✓ 2 tbsp Kalamata olives, chopped
- ✓ ½ tsp dried oregano
- ✓ 2 cups spinach
- ❖ Add the halloumi cheese slices to the grill. Cook for 2 minutes per side or until golden brown marks appear on the grill.
- ❖ In a bowl, mix red peppers, tomatoes, olives, vinegar, oregano, spinach and remaining olive oil; toss to coat. Spread mayonnaise on 4 mushroom "sandwiches", top with a slice of halloumi, a scoop of greens and top with remaining mushrooms. Serve and enjoy!

Nutrition: Calories 339, Fat 29.4g, Net Carbs 3.5g, Protein 10g

195) **Sriracha tofu with yogurt sauce**

Preparation Time: 40 minutes   **Servings: 4**

Ingredients:

- ✓ 12 ounces tofu, pressed and sliced
- ✓ 1 cup green onions, chopped
- ✓ 1 clove garlic, minced
- ✓ 2 tbsp vinegar
- ✓ 1 tbsp sriracha sauce
- ✓ 2 tbsp olive oil

Directions:

- ❖ Place the tofu slices, garlic, sriracha sauce, vinegar and green onions in a bowl. Let stand for 30 minutes. Place a nonstick skillet over medium heat and add oil to heat. Cook the tofu for 5 minutes until golden brown.

Ingredients:

- ✓ Yogurt Sauce
- ✓ 2 cloves garlic, crushed
- ✓ 2 tbsp fresh lemon juice
- ✓ Salt and black pepper to taste
- ✓ 1 tsp fresh dill
- ✓ 1 cup Greek yogurt
- ✓ 1 cucumber, shredded
- ❖ To make the sauce: In a bowl, mix garlic, salt, yogurt, black pepper, lemon juice and dill. Add shredded cucumber while stirring to combine. Serve tofu with a spoonful of yogurt sauce.

Nutrition: Calories 351; Fat: 25.9g, Net Carbohydrates: 8.1g, Protein: 17.5g

SNACK & SIDE DISHES

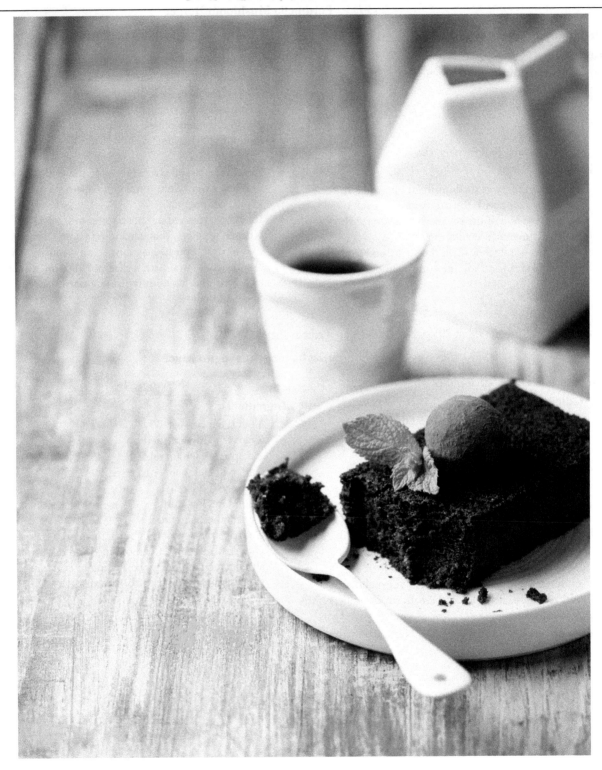

196)   Spinach and Turnip Salad with Bacon

Preparation Time: 40 minutes   **Servings: 4**

Ingredients:

- ✓ 2 turnips, cut into wedges
- ✓ 1 tsp olive oil
- ✓ 1 cup baby spinach, chopped
- ✓ 3 radishes, sliced
- ✓ 3 slices turkey bacon
- ✓ 4 tbsp sour cream

Directions:

- ❖ Preheat oven to 400°F. Line a baking sheet with parchment paper, toss the turnips with salt and black pepper, drizzle with olive oil and bake for 25 minutes, turning halfway through. Allow to cool.

Ingredients:

- ✓ 2 tbsp mustard seed
- ✓ 1 tsp Dijon mustard
- ✓ 1 tbsp red wine vinegar
- ✓ Salt and black pepper to taste
- ✓ 1 tbsp chopped chives

- ❖ Spread the spinach in the bottom of a salad bowl and top with the radishes. Remove the turnips to the salad bowl. Fry the bacon in a skillet over medium heat until crispy, about 5 minutes.
- ❖ Mix sour cream, mustard seeds, mustard, vinegar and salt with the bacon. Add a little water to deglaze the bottom of the pan. Pour the bacon mixture over the vegetables and scatter the chives. Serve.

Nutrition: Calories 193, Fat 18.3g, Net Carbohydrates 3.1g, Protein 9.5g

197)   Chicken Salad with Grapefruit and Cashews

Preparation Time: 30 minutes + marinating time   **Servings: 4**

Ingredients:

- ✓ 1 grapefruit, peeled and segmented
- ✓ 1 chicken breast
- ✓ 4 green onions, sliced
- ✓ 10 ounces baby spinach
- ✓ 2 tbsp cashews

Directions:

- ❖ Toast cashews in a dry skillet over high heat for 2 minutes, shaking often. Set aside to cool, then cut them into small pieces. Preheat the grill to medium heat. Season the chicken with salt and pepper and brush it with a little olive oil.

Ingredients:

- ✓ 1 red chili pepper, thinly sliced
- ✓ 1 lemon, squeezed
- ✓ 3 tbsp olive oil
- ✓ Salt and black pepper to taste

- ❖ Grill for 4 minutes per side. Remove to a plate and let it rest for a few minutes before slicing.
- ❖ Arrange the spinach and green onions on a serving platter. Season with salt, remaining olive oil and lemon juice. Stir to coat. Top with the chicken, chili and chicken. Sprinkle with cashews and serve.

Nutrition: Calories 178, Fat: 13.5g, Net carbohydrates: 3.2g, Protein: 9.1g

198) Cobb Salad with Blue Cheese Dressing

Preparation Time: 30 minutes

Servings: 6

Ingredients:

- ✓ Dressing
- ✓ ½ cup buttermilk
- ✓ 1 cup mayonnaise
- ✓ 2 tbsp Worcestershire sauce
- ✓ ½ cup sour cream
- ✓ 1 cup blue cheese, crumbled
- ✓ 2 tbsp chives, chopped
- ✓ Salad
- ✓ 6 eggs
- ✓ 2 chicken breasts

Directions:

- ❖ In a bowl, whisk buttermilk, mayonnaise, Worcestershire sauce and sour cream. Stir in the blue cheese and chives. Refrigerate to chill until ready to use. Bring eggs to boil in salted water over medium heat for 10 minutes. Transfer to an ice bath to cool. Peel and chop. Set aside.
- ❖ Preheat a grill pan over high heat. Season chicken with salt and pepper. Grill for 3 minutes on each side. Remove to a plate to cool for 3 minutes and cut into pieces.

Ingredients:

- ✓ 5 strips of bacon
- ✓ 1 iceberg lettuce, chopped
- ✓ Salt and black pepper to taste
- ✓ 1 romaine lettuce, cut into pieces
- ✓ 1 bibb lettuce, core, leaves removed
- ✓ 2 avocados, pitted and diced
- ✓ 2 large tomatoes, chopped
- ✓ ½ cup blue cheese, crumbled
- ✓ 2 shallots, chopped

- ❖ . Fry the bacon in the same skillet until crispy, about 6 minutes. Remove, let cool for 2 minutes and cut into pieces.
- ❖ Arrange the lettuce leaves in a salad bowl and, in individual piles, add the avocado, tomatoes, eggs, bacon and chicken. Sprinkle the salad with the blue cheese, scallions and black pepper. Drizzle the blue cheese dressing over the salad and serve with low carb bread.

Nutrition: Calories 122, Fat 14g, Net Carbs 2g, Protein 23g

199) Green mackerel salad

Preparation Time: 25 minutes

Servings: 4

Ingredients:

- ✓ 4 oz smoked mackerel, flaked
- ✓ 2 eggs
- ✓ 1 tbsp coconut oil
- ✓ 1 cup green beans, chopped
- ✓ 1 avocado, sliced

Directions:

- ❖ In a bowl, whisk together the lemon juice, olive oil, salt and pepper. Set aside. Cook green beans in boiling salted water over medium heat for about 3 minutes. Remove with a slotted spoon and let cool.

Ingredients:

- ✓ 4 cups mixed salad
- ✓ 2 tbsp olive oil
- ✓ 1 tbsp lemon juice
- ✓ Salt and black pepper to taste

- ❖ Add the eggs to the pot and cook for 8-10 minutes. Transfer the eggs to an ice water bath, peel the shells and slice. Place the mixed green salad in a serving bowl and add the green beans and smoked mackerel. Pour in the dressing and toss to coat. Top with sliced egg and avocado and serve.

Nutrition: Calories 356, Fat: 31.9g, Net Carbs: 0.8g, Protein: 1.3g

200) **Grilled Steak Salad with Pickled Peppers**

Preparation Time: 15 minutes

Servings: 4

Ingredients:
- ✓ ½ lb skirt steak, sliced
- ✓ Salt and black pepper to taste
- ✓ 3 tbsp olive oil
- ✓ 1 head romaine lettuce, torn

Directions:
- ❖ Brush the steak slices with olive oil and season them with salt and black pepper on both sides. Heat a grill pan over high heat and cook the steaks on each side for about 5-6 minutes. Remove to a bowl.

Ingredients:
- ✓ 3 pickled peppers, chopped
- ✓ 2 tbsp red wine vinegar
- ✓ ½ cup queso fresco, crumbled
- ✓ 1 tbsp green olives, pitted, sliced
- ❖ Mix the lettuce, pickled peppers, remaining olive oil and vinegar in a salad bowl. Add beef and sprinkle with queso fresco and green olives. Serve.

Nutrition: Calories 315, Fat 26g, Net Carbs 2g, Protein 18g

201) **Cauliflower salad with shrimp and avocado**

Preparation Time: 30 minutes

Servings: 6

Ingredients:
- ✓ 1 head cauliflower, florets only
- ✓ 1 pound medium shrimp, shelled
- ✓ ¼ cup + 1 tbsp olive oil
- ✓ 1 avocado, chopped

Directions:
- ❖ Heat 1 tbsp olive oil in a skillet and cook the shrimp for 8 minutes. Microwave the cauliflower for 5 minutes

Ingredients:
- ✓ 2 tbsp fresh dill, chopped
- ✓ ¼ cup lemon juice
- ✓ 2 tbsp lemon zest
- ✓ Salt and black pepper to taste
- ❖ Place the shrimp, cauliflower, and avocado in a bowl. Whisk the remaining olive oil, lemon zest, juice, dill, salt and pepper in another bowl. Pour over the dressing, toss to combine and serve immediately.

Nutrition: Calories 214, Fat: 17g, Net Carbs: 5g, Protein: 15g

202) **Caesar Salad with Smoked Salmon and Poached Eggs**

Preparation Time: 15 minutes

Servings: 4

Ingredients:
- ✓ 8 eggs
- ✓ 2 cups torn romaine lettuce
- ✓ ½ cup smoked salmon, chopped

Directions:
- ❖ Bring a pot of water to a boil and pour in the vinegar. Crack each egg into a small bowl and gently slide it into the water. Soak for 2 to 3 minutes, remove with a slotted spoon and transfer to a paper towel to remove excess water and plate. Poach the remaining 7 eggs.

Ingredients:
- ✓ 6 slices of bacon
- ✓ 2 tbsp low-carb Caesar dressing
- ✓ 1 tbsp white wine vinegar
- ❖ Place the bacon in a skillet and fry it over medium heat until browned and crispy, about 6 minutes, turning once. Remove, let cool and cut into small pieces. Mix the lettuce, smoked salmon, bacon and Caesar dressing in a salad bowl. Top with two eggs each and serve immediately or chilled.

Nutrition: Calories 260, Fat 21g, Net Carbs 5g, Protein 8g

203) **Bacon and Spinach Salad**

Preparation Time: 20 minutes

Servings: 4

Ingredients:
- ✓ 1 avocado, chopped
- ✓ 1 avocado, sliced
- ✓ 1 spring onion, sliced
- ✓ 4 slices bacon, chopped
- ✓ 2 cups spinach
- ✓ 2 small heads of lettuce, chopped

Directions:
- ❖ Place a skillet over medium heat and cook the bacon for 5 minutes until crispy. Remove to a paper towel-lined plate to drain. Boil the eggs in boiling salted water for 10 minutes. Let them cool, peel and chop them.

Ingredients:
- ✓ 2 eggs
- ✓ 3 tbsp olive oil
- ✓ 1 tbsp Dijon mustard
- ✓ 1 tbsp apple cider vinegar
- ✓ Salt to taste

- ❖ Combine the spinach, lettuce, eggs, chopped avocado and spring onion in a large bowl. Whisk together the olive oil, mustard, apple cider vinegar and salt in another bowl. Pour the dressing over the salad and toss to combine. Top with the sliced avocado and bacon and serve.

Nutrition: Calories 350, Fat: 33g, Net Carbs: 3.4g, Protein: 7g

204) **Brussels Sprouts Salad with Pecorino Cheese**

Preparation Time: 35 minutes

Servings: 6

Ingredients:
- ✓ 2 lb Brussels sprouts, halved
- ✓ 3 tbsp olive oil
- ✓ Salt and black pepper to taste

Directions:
- ❖ Preheat the oven to 400°F. Toss brussels sprouts with olive oil, salt, black pepper and balsamic vinegar in a bowl. Spread on a baking sheet in an even layer.

Ingredients:
- ✓ 2 tbsp balsamic vinegar
- ✓ ¼ head red cabbage, shredded
- ✓ 1 cup Pecorino cheese, shredded
- ❖ Bake until tender on the inside and crisp on the outside, about 20-25 minutes. Transfer to a salad bowl and add the red cabbage. Stir until well combined. Sprinkle with cheese, divide salad on serving plates and serve.

Nutrition: Calories 210, Fat 18g, Net Carbs 6g, Protein 4g

205) **Pork Burger Salad with Yellow Cheddar**

Preparation Time: 25 minutes

Servings: 4

Ingredients:
- ✓ ½ pound ground pork
- ✓ Salt and black pepper to taste
- ✓ 2 tbsp olive oil
- ✓ 2 hearts of romaine lettuce, torn

Directions:
- ❖ Season the pork with salt and black pepper, mix it, and make medium-sized patties. Heat the butter in a skillet over medium heat and fry the patties on both sides for 10 minutes until golden brown and cooked through on the inside.

Ingredients:
- ✓ 2 firm tomatoes, sliced
- ✓ ¼ red onion, sliced
- ✓ 3 ounces yellow cheddar cheese, grated
- ✓ 2 tbsp butter
- ❖ Transfer to a rack to drain off the oil. Once cooled, cut into quarters.
- ❖ Mix the lettuce, tomatoes, and red onion in a salad bowl, drizzle with olive oil and salt. Stir and add the pork on top. Top with cheese and serve.

Nutrition: Calories 310, Fat 23g, Net Carbs 2g, Protein 22g

206) **Italian style green salad**

Preparation Time: 15 minutes

Ingredients:

- ✓ 2 (8 oz) package mixed salad
- ✓ 8 strips of bacon
- ✓ 1 cup gorgonzola cheese, crumbled

Directions:

- ❖ Fry the bacon strips in a skillet over medium heat for 6 minutes, until golden brown and crispy. Remove to a paper towel-lined plate to drain. Chop when cooled. Pour the green salad into a serving bowl.

Nutrition: Calories 205, Fat 20g, Net Carbs 2g, Protein 4g

Servings: 4

Ingredients:

- ✓ 1 tbsp white wine vinegar
- ✓ 3 tbsp extra virgin olive oil
- ✓ Salt and black pepper to taste
- ❖ In a small bowl, whisk the white wine vinegar, olive oil, salt and pepper. Drizzle the dressing over the salad and toss to coat. Top with gorgonzola cheese and bacon. Divide salad among plates and serve.

207) **Broccoli Salad Salad with Mustard Vinaigrette**

Preparation Time: 10 minutes

Ingredients:

- ✓ ½ tsp granulated sugar swerve
- ✓ 1 tbsp Dijon mustard
- ✓ 2 tbsp olive oil
- ✓ 4 cups broccoli salad
- ✓ ⅓ cup mayonnaise

Directions:

- ❖ In a bowl, place the mayonnaise, Dijon mustard, sugar swerve, olive oil, celery seeds, vinegar and salt and whisk until well combined.

Nutrition: Calories 110, Fat: 10g, Net Carbs: 2g, Protein: 3g

Servings: 6

Ingredients:

- ✓ 1 tsp celery seeds
- ✓ 2 tbsp slivered almonds
- ✓ 1 ½ tbsp apple cider vinegar
- ✓ Salt to taste

- ❖ Place the broccoli salad in a large salad bowl. Pour the vinaigrette over the top. Stir to coat. Sprinkle with slivered almonds and serve immediately.

208) **Warm Artichoke Salad**

Preparation Time: 30 minutes

Ingredients:

- ✓ 6 baby artichokes
- ✓ 6 cups water
- ✓ 1 tbsp lemon juice
- ✓ ¼ cup cherry peppers, halved
- ✓ ¼ cup pitted olives, sliced
- ✓ ¼ cup olive oil

Directions:

- ❖ Combine the water and salt in a saucepan over medium heat. Trim and halve the artichokes. Add them to the pot and bring to a boil. Lower the heat and simmer for 20 minutes until tender.

Nutrition: Calories 170, Fat: 13g, Net carbs: 5g, Protein: 1g

Servings: 4

Ingredients:

- ✓ ¼ tsp lemon zest
- ✓ 2 tbsp balsamic vinegar, unsweetened
- ✓ 1 tbsp chopped dill
- ✓ Salt and black pepper to taste
- ✓ 1 tbsp capers
- ✓ ¼ tsp caper brine
- ❖ Combine the rest of the ingredients, except the olives, in a bowl. Drain and arrange the artichokes on a serving platter. Pour prepared mixture over them; toss to combine well. Serve topped with the olives.

209) **Squid salad with cucumbers and chili sauce**

Preparation Time: 30 minutes

Servings: 4

Ingredients:
- ✓ 4 tubes of squid, cut into strips
- ✓ ½ cup mint leaves
- ✓ 2 cucumbers, halved, cut into strips
- ✓ ½ cup cilantro, stalks reserved
- ✓ ½ red onion, finely sliced
- ✓ Salt and black pepper to taste

Directions:
- ❖ In a salad bowl, mix mint leaves, cucumber strips, cilantro leaves and red onion. Season with salt, black pepper and a little olive oil; set aside. In a mortar, pound the cilantro stalks and red pepper to form a paste using the pestle. Add the fish sauce and lime juice and stir with the pestle.

Ingredients:
- ✓ 1 tsp fish sauce
- ✓ 1 red chili pepper, coarsely chopped
- ✓ 1 garlic clove
- ✓ 2 limes, squeezed
- ✓ 1 tbsp fresh parsley, chopped
- ✓ 1 tsp olive oil

- ❖ Heat a frying pan over medium heat. Brown the squid on both sides until lightly browned, about 5 minutes. Pour the calamari over the salad and drizzle with the chili dressing. Stir to coat, garnish with parsley and serve.

Nutrition: Calories 318, Fat 22.5g, Net Carbohydrates 2.1g, Protein 24.6g

210) **Mozzarella and tomato salad with anchovies and olives**

Preparation Time: 10 minutes

Servings: 2

Ingredients:
- ✓ 1 large tomato, sliced
- ✓ 4 basil leaves
- ✓ 8 slices of mozzarella
- ✓ 2 tbsp olive oil

Directions:
- ❖ Arrange the tomato slices on a serving platter. Place the mozzarella slices on top and top with the basil.

Ingredients:
- ✓ 2 canned anchovies, chopped
- ✓ 1 tsp balsamic vinegar
- ✓ 4 black olives, pitted and sliced
- ✓ Salt to taste
- ❖ Add the anchovies and olives on top. Drizzle with olive oil and vinegar. Sprinkle with salt and serve.

Nutrition: Calories 430, Fat: 26.8g, Net Carbohydrates: 2.4g, Protein:38.8g

211) **Strawberry salad with cheese and almonds**

Preparation Time: 20 minutes

Servings: 2

Ingredients:
- ✓ 4 cups cabbage, chopped
- ✓ 4 strawberries, sliced
- ✓ ½ cup almonds, slivered

Directions:
- ❖ Preheat oven to 400°F. Arrange grated goat cheese in two circles on two pieces of parchment paper. Place in the oven and bake for 10 minutes. Find two equal bowls, place them upside down and carefully place the parchment paper on top to give the cheese a bowl-like shape.

Ingredients:
- ✓ 1 ½ cups hard goat cheese, grated
- ✓ 4 tbsp raspberry vinaigrette
- ✓ Salt and black pepper to taste
- ❖ Let cool like this for 15 minutes.
- ❖ Divide the cabbage between the bowls, sprinkle with salt and pepper, and drizzle with the vinaigrette. Stir to coat. Top with almonds and strawberries. Serve immediately.

Nutrition: Calories 445, Fat: 34.2g, Net Carbohydrates: 5.3g, Protein: 33g

212) **Spring salad with cheese balls**

Preparation Time: 20 minutes

Ingredients:
- ✓ Cheese balls
- ✓ 3 eggs
- ✓ 1 cup feta cheese, crumbled
- ✓ ½ cup Pecorino cheese, crumbled
- ✓ 1 cup Almond Flour
- ✓ 1 tbsp flax meal
- ✓ Salt and black pepper to taste
- ✓ Salad
- ✓ 1 head Iceberg lettuce, leaves pulled apart
- ✓ ½ cup cucumber, thinly sliced

Directions:
- ❖ Preheat oven to 390°F. In a bowl, mix all the ingredients for the cheese balls. Form balls with the mixture. Place the balls on a lined baking sheet. Bake for 10 minutes until crispy.

Servings: 6

Ingredients:
- ✓ 2 tomatoes, seeded and chopped
- ✓ ½ cup red onion, thinly sliced
- ✓ ½ cup radishes, thinly sliced
- ✓ ⅓ cup mayonnaise
- ✓ 1 tsp mustard
- ✓ 1 tsp paprika
- ✓ 1 tsp oregano
- ✓ Salt to taste

- ❖ Arrange lettuce leaves on a large salad plate. Add radishes, tomatoes, cucumbers and red onion. In a small bowl, mix mayonnaise, paprika, salt, oregano and mustard. Sprinkle the mixture over the vegetables. Add cheese balls on top and serve.

Nutrition: Calories: 234; Fat 16.7g, Net Carbohydrates 7.9g, Protein 12.4g

213) **Mediterranean Salad**

Preparation Time: 10 minutes

Ingredients:
- ✓ 3 tomatoes, sliced
- ✓ 1 large avocado, sliced
- ✓ 8 kalamata olives

Directions:
- ❖ Arrange the tomato slices on a serving platter and place the avocado slices in the center.

Servings: 4

Ingredients:
- ✓ ¼ lb buffalo mozzarella, sliced
- ✓ 2 tbsp pesto sauce
- ✓ 1 tbsp olive oil
- ❖ Arrange the olives around the avocado slices and drop mozzarella pieces onto the serving plate. Drizzle the pesto sauce and olive oil over everything and serve.

Nutrition: Calories 290, Fat: 25g, Net carbs: 4.3g, Protein: 9g

214) **Tuna salad with lettuce and olives**

Preparation Time: 5 minutes

Ingredients:
- ✓ 1 cup canned tuna, drained
- ✓ 1 tsp of onion flakes
- ✓ 3 tbsp mayonnaise

Directions:
- ❖ Combine tuna, mayonnaise and lime juice in a small bowl. Stir to combine. In a salad bowl, arrange shredded lettuce and onion flakes.

Servings: 2

Ingredients:
- ✓ 1 cup romaine lettuce, shredded
- ✓ 1 tbsp lime juice
- ✓ 6 black olives, pitted and sliced
- ❖ Spread the tuna mixture over the top. Top with black olives and serve.

Nutrition: Calories 248, Fat: 20g, Net Carbs: 2g, Protein: 18.5g

215) Cobb egg salad in lettuce cups

Preparation Time: 25 minutes

Servings: 4

Ingredients:

- ✓ 1 head of green lettuce, firm leaves removed for cups
- ✓ 2 chicken breasts, cut into pieces
- ✓ 1 tbsp olive oil
- ✓ Salt and black pepper to taste

Directions:

- ❖ Preheat oven to 400°F. Place chicken in a bowl, drizzle with olive oil and sprinkle with salt and black pepper. Cough to coat. Place the chicken on a baking sheet and spread it out evenly. Slide the baking sheet into the oven and bake the chicken until cooked through and golden brown for 8 minutes, stirring once.

Ingredients:

- ✓ 6 large eggs
- ✓ 2 tomatoes, seeded, chopped
- ✓ 6 tbsp Greek yogurt

- ❖ Boil the eggs in salted water for 10 minutes. Allow them to cool, peel and cut into pieces. Transfer to a salad bowl. Remove the chicken from the oven and add it to the salad bowl. Include the tomatoes and Greek yogurt and toss to combine. Layer 2 lettuce leaves each as cups and fill with 2 tbsp of egg salad each. Serve.

Nutrition: Calories 325, Fat 24.5g, Net Carbs 4g, Protein 21g

216) Waffle sandwiches with gruyere and ham

Preparation Time: 20 minutes

Servings: 4

Ingredients:

- ✓ 4 slices smoked ham, chopped
- ✓ 4 tbsp butter, softened
- ✓ ½ cup Gruyere cheese, grated
- ✓ 6 eggs

Directions:

- ❖ In a bowl, mix the eggs, baking powder, thyme and butter. Place a waffle iron over medium heat, add ¼ cup of the batter and cook for 6 minutes until golden brown. Do the same with the remaining batter until you have 8 thin waffles.

Ingredients:

- ✓ ½ tsp baking powder
- ✓ ½ tsp dried thyme
- ✓ 4 slices tomato

- ❖ Lay a slice of tomato on one waffle, followed by a slice of ham, then top with ¼ of the grated cheese. Cover with another waffle, place the sandwich in the waffle iron and cook until the cheese melts. Repeat with remaining ingredients.

Nutrition: Calories 276; Net carbs 3.1g; Fat 22g; Protein 16g

217) Baked chorizo with ricotta cheese

Preparation Time: 30 minutes

Servings: 6

Ingredients:

- ✓ 7 ounces Spanish chorizo, sliced
- ✓ 4 ounces ricotta cheese, crumbled

Directions:

- ❖ Preheat oven to 325 F. Spread chorizo on a wax paper-lined baking sheet and bake for 15 minutes until crispy

Ingredients:

- ✓ ¼ cup chopped parsley

- ❖ Remove from oven and allow to cool. Arrange on a serving platter. Add ricotta cheese and parsley.

Nutrition: Calories 172; Net carbohydrates: 0.2g; Fat: 13g; Protein: 5g

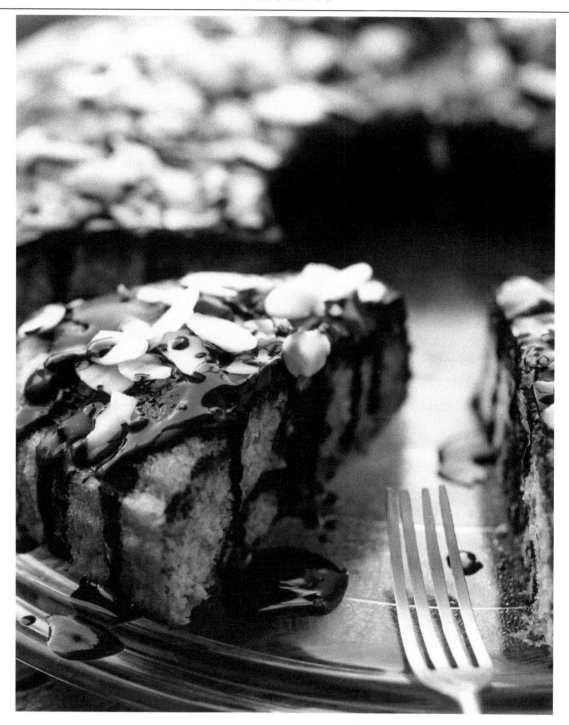

218) Coconut fat bombs

Preparation Time: 2 minutes + cooling time

Servings: 4

Ingredients:
- ✓ 2/3 cup coconut oil, melted
- ✓ 1 can of coconut milk (14 ounces)

Directions:
- ❖ Mix the coconut oil with the milk and stevia. Stir in coconut flakes until well distributed.

Ingredients:
- ✓ 18 drops of liquid stevia
- ✓ 1 cup unsweetened coconut flakes
- ❖ Pour into silicone muffin molds and freeze for 1 hour to harden.

Nutrition: Calories 214, fat 19g, net carbs 2g, protein 4g

219) Dark Chocolate Mochaccino Ice Bombs

Preparation Time: 5 minutes + cooling time

Servings: 4

Ingredients:
- ✓ ½ pound of cream cheese
- ✓ 4 tbsp powdered sweetener
- ✓ 2 ounces of strong coffee

Directions:
- ❖ Combine the cream cheese, sweetener, coffee and cocoa powder in a food processor. Spread 2 tbsp of the mixture and place on a lined tray.

Ingredients:
- ✓ 2 tbsp unsweetened cocoa powder
- ✓ 1 tbsp cocoa butter, melted
- ✓ 2 1/2 ounces melted dark chocolate
- ❖ . Mix in the melted cocoa butter and chocolate and coat the bombs with it. Freeze for 2 hours.

Nutrition: Calories Calories 127, Fat: 13g, Net Carbohydrates: 1.4g, Protein: 1.9g

220) Strawberry and ricotta parfait

Preparation Time: 10 minutes

Servings: 4

Ingredients:
- ✓ 2 cups strawberries, chopped
- ✓ 1 cup ricotta cheese

Directions:
- ❖ Divide half of the strawberries among 4 small glasses and top with the ricotta.

Ingredients:
- ✓ 2 tbsp sugar-free maple syrup
- ✓ 2 tbsp balsamic vinegar
- ❖ Drizzle with maple syrup, balsamic vinegar and finish with remaining strawberries. Serve.

Nutrition: Calories 164; Net carbs 3.1g; Fat 8.2g; Protein 7g

221) Creamy strawberry mousse

Preparation Time: 10 minutes + cooling time

Servings:

Ingredients:
- ✓ 2 cups frozen strawberries
- ✓ 2 tbsp sugar swerve

Directions:
- ❖ Pour 1 ½ cups of strawberries into a blender and process until smooth. Add the swerve sugar and process further. Pour in the egg whites and transfer the mixture to a bowl.

Ingredients:
- ✓ 1 large egg white
- ✓ 2 cups whipped cream
- ❖ Use an electric hand whisk to beat until the mixture is frothy. Pour mixture into dessert glasses and top with whipped cream and strawberries. Serve chilled.

Nutrition: Calories 145; Net carbohydrates 4.8g; Fat 6.8g; Protein 2g

222) **Berry Clafoutis**

Preparation Time: 45 minutes

Servings: 4

Ingredients:

- ✓ 4 eggs
- ✓ 2 tbsp coconut oil
- ✓ 2 cups berries
- ✓ 1 cup coconut milk

Ingredients:

- ✓ 1 cup almond flour
- ✓ ¼ cup sweetener
- ✓ ½ tsp vanilla powder
- ✓ 1 tbsp powdered sweetener
- ❖ Gently add the berries. Grease a flan pan with coconut oil and pour in the mixture. Bake for 35 minutes. Sprinkle with powdered sugar and serve.

Directions:

- ❖ Preheat oven to 350 F. Place all ingredients except coconut oil, berries and sweetener powder in a blender until smooth.

Nutrition: Calories 198; Net carbs 4.9g; Fat 16g; Protein 15g

223) **Coconut and raspberry cheesecake**

Preparation Time: 40 minutes + cooling time

Servings: 6

Ingredients:

- ✓ 2 egg whites
- ✓ 1 ¼ cups erythritol
- ✓ 3 cups desiccated coconut
- ✓ 1 tbsp coconut oil
- ✓ ¼ cup melted butter

Ingredients:

- ✓ 3 tbsp lemon juice
- ✓ 6 ounces raspberries
- ✓ 1 cup whipped cream
- ✓ 3 tbsp lemon juice
- ✓ 24 ounces of cream cheese
- ❖ Add lemon juice and remaining erythritol. In another bowl, beat the heavy cream with an electric mixer. Fold the whipped cream into the cream cheese mixture; stir in the raspberries. Spread the filling over the baked crust. Refrigerate for 4 hours. Serve.

Directions:

- ❖ Preheat oven to 350 F. Grease a baking sheet with coconut oil and line with baking paper. Mix egg whites, ¼ cup erythritol, coconut and butter until a crust forms and pour into the baking dish. Bake for 25 minutes. Allow to cool. Beat the cream cheese until smooth.

Nutrition: Calories 215; Net Carbs 3g; Fat 25g; Protein 5g

224) **Peanut butter and chocolate ice cream bars**

Preparation Time: approxi 4 hours and 20 minutes

Servings: 6

Ingredients:

- ✓ ¼ cup cocoa butter chunks, chopped
- ✓ 2 cups heavy whipping cream
- ✓ ⅔ cup peanut butter, softened
- ✓ 1 ½ cups almond milk

Ingredients:

- ✓ 1 tbsp vegetable glycerin
- ✓ 6 tbsp xylitol
- ✓ ¾ cup coconut oil
- ✓ 2 ounces unsweetened chocolate
- ❖ Mix coconut oil, cocoa butter, chocolate and remaining xylitol and microwave until melted; let cool slightly. Cut ice cream into bars. Dip into chocolate mixture. Serve.

Directions:

- ❖ Mix the heavy cream, peanut butter, almond milk, vegetable glycerin and half of the xylitol until smooth. Place in an ice cream maker and follow instructions. Spread the ice cream into a lined baking dish and freeze for 4 hours.

Nutrition: Calories 345 Net carbohydrates 5g; Fat 32g; Protein 4g

225) Lemon and yogurt mousse

Preparation Time: 5 minutes + cooling time

Servings:

Ingredients:

- ✓ 24 ounces plain yogurt, strained overnight in cheesecloth
- ✓ 2 cups powdered sugar swerve

Ingredients:

- ✓ 2 lemons, squeezed and peeled
- ✓ 1 cup whipped cream + extra for garnish

Directions:

- ❖ Whip plain yogurt in a bowl with a hand mixer until light and fluffy. Stir in the swerve sugar, lemon juice and salt. Add the whipped cream to combine.

- ❖ Pour mousse into serving cups and refrigerate for 1 hour. Swirl with more whipped cream and garnish with lemon zest.

Nutrition: Calories 223; Net Carbs 3g; Fat 18g; Protein 12g

226) Strawberry Chocolate Mousse

Preparation Time: 30 minutes

Servings: 4

Ingredients:

- ✓ 1 cup fresh strawberries, sliced
- ✓ 3 eggs
- ✓ 1 cup dark chocolate chips

Ingredients:

- ✓ 1 cup heavy cream
- ✓ 1 vanilla extract
- ✓ 1 tbsp sugar swerve
- ❖ Whisk in the eggs, vanilla extract and sugar swerve. Add the cooled chocolate. Divide the mousse between glasses, top with the strawberry and chill in the refrigerator. Serve.

Directions:

- ❖ Melt chocolate in a microwave-safe bowl in the microwave for 1 minute; let cool for 8 minutes. In a bowl, whip heavy cream until very smooth.

Nutrition: Calories 400; Net Carbs 1.7g; Fat 25g; Protein 8g

227) Maple Lemon Cake

Preparation Time: 30 minutes

Servings:

Ingredients:

- ✓ 4 eggs
- ✓ 1 cup sour cream
- ✓ 2 lemons, peeled and squeezed
- ✓ 1 tsp vanilla extract
- ✓ 2 cups almond flour
- ✓ 2 tbsp coconut flour

Ingredients:

- ✓ 2 tbsp baking powder
- ✓ ½ cup xylitol
- ✓ 1 tsp cardamom powder
- ✓ ½ tsp ground ginger
- ✓ A pinch of salt
- ✓ ¼ cup maple syrup

Directions:

- ❖ Preheat oven to 400 F. Grease a cake pan with melted butter. In a bowl, beat the eggs, sour cream, lemon juice and vanilla extract until smooth. In another bowl, whisk together the almond and coconut flours, baking powder, xylitol, cardamom, ginger, salt, lemon zest and half of the maple syrup.

- ❖ Combine both mixtures until smooth and pour the batter into the baking dish. Bake for 25 minutes or until a toothpick inserted comes out clean. Transfer to a wire rack, let cool and drizzle with remaining maple syrup. Serve in slices.

Nutrition: Calories 441; Net Carbs 8.5g; Fat 29g; Protein 33g

228) Flan with whipped cream

Preparation Time: 10 minutes + cooling time

Servings: 4

Ingredients:

- ✓ ⅓ cup erythritol, for the caramel
- ✓ 2 cups almond milk
- ✓ 4 eggs
- ✓ 1 tbsp vanilla

Ingredients:

- ✓ 1 tbsp lemon zest
- ✓ ½ cup erythritol, for the custard
- ✓ 2 cups heavy whipping cream
- ✓ Mint leaves, for serving
- ❖ Pour enough hot water into the baking dish to halfway up the sides of the cups. Bake at 345 F for 45 minutes. Remove the ramekins and place them in the refrigerator for 4 hours. Take a knife and run slowly around the edges to spill onto plates. Serve with spoonfuls of cream and mint leaves.

Directions:

- ❖ Heat the erythritol for the caramel in a pan. Add 2-3 tbsp of water and bring to a boil. Reduce heat and cook until caramel turns golden brown. Carefully divide among 4 metal cups. Allow them to cool. In a bowl, mix the eggs, remaining erythritol, lemon zest and vanilla. Add the almond milk and beat again until combined. Pour the cream into the caramel lined cups and place in a baking dish.

Nutrition: Calories 169; Net carbs 1.7g; Fat 10g; Protein 7g

229) Chocolate and walnut cookies

Preparation Time: 30 minutes

Servings: 4

Ingredients:

- ✓ 2/3 cup dark chocolate chips
- ✓ 4 ounces butter, softened
- ✓ 2 tbsp swerve sugar
- ✓ 2 tbsp brown sugar swerve
- ✓ 1 egg

Ingredients:

- ✓ 1 tsp vanilla extract
- ✓ ½ cup almond flour
- ✓ ½ tsp baking soda
- ✓ ½ cup chopped walnuts
- ❖ Spoon full tbsp of batter onto a greased baking sheet, leaving 2 inches of space between each spoonful. Press each batter to flatten slightly. Bake for 15 minutes. Transfer to a rack to cool completely. Serve.

Directions:

- ❖ Preheat oven to 350 F. In a bowl, beat butter, swerve sugar and swerve brown sugar until smooth. Beat in the egg and stir in the vanilla extract. In another bowl, combine the almond flour with the baking soda and mix into the wet ingredients. Add the chocolate chips and walnuts.

Nutrition: Calories 430; Net carbohydrates 3.5g; Fat 42g; Protein 6g

230) Quick Blueberry Sorbet

Preparation Time: 15 minutes + cooling time

Servings: 4

Ingredients:

- ✓ 4 cups frozen blueberries
- ✓ 1 cup sugar swerve

Ingredients:

- ✓ ½ lemon, squeezed
- ✓ ½ tsp salt
- ❖ Chill for 3 hours. Pour cooled juice into an ice cream maker and strain until mixture resembles ice cream. Spoon into a bowl and chill further for 3 hours.

Directions:

- ❖ In a blender, add blueberries, swerve, lemon juice and salt; process until smooth. Strain through a strainer into a bowl.

Nutrition: Calories 178; Net Carbs 2.3g; Fat 1g; Protein 0.6g

231)   **Trifle of mixed berries**

Preparation Time: 3 minutes + cooling time

Servings: 4

Ingredients:
- ✓ ½ cup walnuts, toasted
- ✓ 1 avocado, chopped
- ✓ 1 cup mascarpone cheese, softened

Directions:
- ❖ In four dessert glasses, divide half of the mascarpone, half of the berries (mixed), half of the walnuts and half of the avocado.

Ingredients:
- ✓ 1 cup fresh blueberries
- ✓ 1 cup fresh raspberries
- ✓ 1 cup fresh blackberries
- ❖ Repeat the layering process a second time to finish the ingredients. Cover the glasses with plastic wrap and refrigerate for 45 minutes until fairly firm.

Nutrition: Calories 321, Fat 28.5g, Net Carbohydrates 8.3g, Protein 9.8g

232)   **Creamy Coconut Kiwi Drink**

Preparation Time: 3 minutes

Servings: 4

Ingredients:
- ✓ 5 kiwis, picked pulp
- ✓ 2 tbsp of erythritol
- ✓ 2 cups unsweetened coconut milk

Directions:
- ❖ In a blender, process the kiwis, erythritol, milk, cream and ice cubes until smooth, about 3 minutes.

Ingredients:
- ✓ 2 cups of coconut cream
- ✓ 7 ice cubes
- ✓ Mint leaves for garnish
- ❖ Pour into four serving glasses, garnish with mint leaves and serve.

Nutrition: Calories 351, Fat 28g, Net Carbs 9.7g, Protein 16g

233)   **Walnut Cookies**

Preparation Time: 15 minutes

Servings: 12

Ingredients:
- ✓ 1 egg
- ✓ 2 cups ground pecans
- ✓ ¼ cup sweetener

Directions:
- ❖ Preheat oven to 350°F. Mix ingredients, except walnuts, until combined. Make 20 balls with the dough and press them with your thumb onto a lined cookie sheet.

Ingredients:
- ✓ ½ tsp baking soda
- ✓ 1 tbsp butter
- ✓ 20 walnut halves
- ❖ Top each cookie with a walnut half. Bake for about 12 minutes.

Nutrition: Calories 101, Fat: 11g, Net Carbs: 0.6g, Protein: 1.6g

234) Chocolate Bark with Almonds

Preparation Time: 5 minutes + cooling time

Servings: 12

Ingredients:

- ✓ ½ cup toasted almonds, chopped
- ✓ ½ cup butter
- ✓ 10 drops of stevia

Ingredients:

- ✓ ¼ tsp salt
- ✓ ½ cup unsweetened coconut flakes
- ✓ 4 ounces dark chocolate
- ❖ Scatter the almonds on top, coconut flakes and sprinkle with salt. Place in the refrigerator for 1 hour.

Directions:

- ❖ Melt the butter and chocolate together, in the microwave, for 90 seconds. Remove and stir in the stevia. Line a cookie sheet with wax paper and spread the chocolate evenly.

Nutrition: Calories 161, Fat: 15.3g, Net Carbohydrates: 1.9g, Protein: 1.9g

235) Raspberry Sorbet

Preparation Time: 10 minutes + cooling time

Servings: 1

Ingredients:

- ✓ ¼ tsp vanilla extract
- ✓ 1 package of gelatin, unsweetened
- ✓ 1 tbsp heavy whipping cream

Ingredients:

- ✓ 2 tbsp raspberry puree
- ✓ 1 ½ cups crushed ice
- ❖ Add remaining ingredients and ⅓ cup cold water. Blend until smooth and freeze for at least 2 hours.

Directions:

- ❖ Cover gelatin with cold water in a small bowl. Allow to dissolve for 5 minutes. Transfer to a blender.

Nutrition: Calories 173, Fat: 10g, Net Carbohydrates: 3.7g, Protein: 4g

236) Wonderful berry pudding

Preparation Time: 45 minutes

Servings: 2

Ingredients:

- ✓ 1 cup almond flour
- ✓ 2 tbsp of lemon juice
- ✓ 2 cups blueberries
- ✓ 2 tbsp baking powder
- ✓ ½ tsp ground nutmeg
- ✓ ½ cup coconut milk
- ✓ 3 tbsp stevia

Ingredients:

- ✓ 1 tbsp flax meal mixed with 1 tbsp water
- ✓ 3 tbsp melted ghee
- ✓ 1 tbsp vanilla extract
- ✓ 1 tbsp arrowroot powder
- ✓ 1 cup cold water

Directions:

- ❖ In a greased heatproof dish, mix blueberries and lemon juice, stir a little and spread over the bottom.
- ❖ In a bowl, mix flour with nutmeg, stevia, baking powder, vanilla, ghee, flaxseed meal, arrowroot and milk, mix well again and spread over blueberries.

- ❖ Put the water in the Instant Pot, add the trivet and heatproof dish, cover and cook on high heat for 35 minutes.
- ❖ Let pudding cool, transfer to dessert bowls and serve.

Nutrition: Calories 220 | Fat: 4g | Carbohydrates: 9g | Protein: 6g | Fiber: 4g | Sugar: 2g

237)   Orange Dessert

Preparation Time: 45 minutes

Ingredients:
- 1 ¾ cups water
- 1 tsp baking powder
- 1 cup coconut flour
- 2 tbsp stevia
- ½ tbsp cinnamon powder
- 3 tbsp coconut oil, melted

Directions:
- ❖ In a bowl, mix flour with stevia, baking powder, cinnamon, 2 tbsp oil, milk, pecans and raisins; stir and transfer to a greased heatproof dish.
- ❖ Heat a small skillet over medium-high heat, mix ¾ cup water with the orange juice, orange zest and the rest of the oil, stir, bring to a boil and pour over the pecan mixture.

Servings: 2

Ingredients:
- ½ cup coconut milk
- ½ cup pecans, chopped
- ½ cup raisins
- ½ cup orange peel, grated
- ¾ cup orange juice

- ❖ Place 1 cup of water in the Instant Pot, add the heatproof dish, cover and cook on High for 30 minutes.
- ❖ Serve cold.

Nutrition: Calories 142 | Fat: 3g | Carbohydrates: 3g | Protein: 3g | Fiber: 1g | Sugar: 1g

238)   Great Pumpkin Dessert

Preparation Time: 40 minutes

Ingredients:
- 1 and ½ tsp baking powder
- 2 cups of coconut flour
- ½ tsp baking soda
- ¼ tsp ground nutmeg
- 1 tsp cinnamon powder
- ¼ tsp ginger, grated
- 1 cup water

Directions:
- ❖ In a bowl, flour with baking powder, baking soda, cinnamon, ginger, nutmeg, oil, egg white, ghee, vanilla extract, pumpkin puree, stevia and lemon juice, mix well and transfer this to a greased cake pan.

Servings: 2

Ingredients:
- 1 tbsp coconut oil, melted
- 1 egg white
- 1 tbsp vanilla extract
- 1 cup pumpkin puree
- 2 tbsp stevia
- 1 tbsp lemon juice

- ❖ Put the water in the Instant Pot, add the trivet, add the cake pan, cover and bake on High for 30 minutes.
- ❖ Allow cake to cool, cut and serve.

Nutrition: Calories 180 | Fat: 3g | Carbohydrates: 3g | Protein: 4g | Fiber: 2g | Sugar: 0g

239) **Merry Berry**

Preparation Time: 6 minutes

Ingredients:
- ✓ 1 cup strawberries + extra for garnish
- ✓ 1 ½ cups blackberries
- ✓ 1 cup blueberries

Directions:
- ❖ For extra strawberries for garnish, make a single deep cut on their sides; set aside. Add blackberries, strawberries, blueberries, beets and ice cubes to smoothie maker.

Servings: 4

Ingredients:
- ✓ 2 small beets, peeled and chopped
- ✓ 2/3 cup ice cubes
- ✓ 1 lime, squeezed
- ❖ Blend ingredients on high speed until smooth and frothy, about 60 seconds. Add the lime juice and blend for 30 seconds more. Pour the drink into tall smoothie glasses, secure the reserved strawberries on the rim of each glass, stick a straw in and serve the drink immediately.

Nutrition: Calories 83, Fat 3g, Net Carbs 8g, Protein 2.7g

240) **Cinnamon Cookies**

Preparation Time: 25 minutes

Ingredients:
- ✓ Cookies
- ✓ 2 cups almond flour
- ✓ ½ tsp baking soda
- ✓ ¾ cup sweetener
- ✓ ½ cup butter, softened

Directions:
- ❖ Preheat oven to 350°F. Combine all cookie ingredients in a bowl. Make 16 balls with the dough and flatten them with your hands. Combine the cinnamon and erythritol.

Servings: 4

Ingredients:
- ✓ A pinch of salt
- ✓ Coating
- ✓ 2 tbsp erythritol sweetener
- ✓ 1 tsp cinnamon

- ❖ Dip the cookies into the cinnamon mixture and place them on a lined baking sheet. Bake for 15 minutes, until crispy.

Nutrition: Calories 134, Fat: 13g, Net Carbs: 1.5g, Protein: 3g

241) **Vanilla Frappuccino**

Preparation Time: 6 minutes

Ingredients:
- ✓ 3 cups unsweetened vanilla almond milk, chilled Unsweetened chocolate chips for garnish
- ✓ 2 tbsp sugar swerve
- ✓ 1 ½ cups heavy cream, chilled

Directions:
- ❖ Combine almond milk, swerve sugar, heavy cream, vanilla bean and xanthan gum in blender and process on high speed for 1 minute until smooth.

Servings: 4

Ingredients:
- ✓ 1 vanilla bean
- ✓ ¼ tsp xanthan gum

- ❖ Pour into tall shake glasses, sprinkle with chocolate chips and serve immediately.

Nutrition: Calories 193, Fat 14g, Net Carbs 6g, Protein 15g

242) Peanut Butter Pecan Ice Cream

Preparation Time: 36 minutes + cooling time

Servings: 4

Ingredients:

- ✓ ½ cup swerve confectioners sweetener
- ✓ 2 cups heavy cream
- ✓ 1 tbsp of erythritol
- ✓ ½ cup plain peanut butter

Directions:

- ❖ Heat the heavy cream with the peanut butter, olive oil and erythritol in a small skillet over low heat without boiling for about 3 minutes. Remove from heat. In a bowl, beat egg yolks until creamy.

Ingredients:

- ✓ 1 tbsp olive oil
- ✓ 2 egg yolks
- ✓ ½ cup pecans, chopped

- ❖ Stir the eggs into the cream mixture. Continue stirring until a thick batter has formed, about 3 minutes. Pour the cream mixture into a bowl. Place in the refrigerator for 30 minutes. Stir in confectioners' sweetener.
- ❖ Pour mixture into ice cream maker and churn according to manufacturer's instructions. Stir in pecan later and spoon mixture into baking dish. Freeze for 2 hours before serving.

Nutrition: Calories 302, Fat 32g, Net Carbs 2g, Protein 5g

243) Coffee Fat Bombs

Preparation Time: 3 minutes + cooling time

Servings: 6

Ingredients:

- ✓ 6 tbsp prepared coffee at room temperature
- ✓ 1 ½ cups mascarpone cheese
- ✓ ½ cup melted butter

Directions:

- ❖ Beat mascarpone, butter, cocoa powder, erythritol and coffee with a hand mixer until creamy and fluffy, about 1 minute.

Nutrition: Calories 145, fat 14g, net carbs 2g, protein 4g

Ingredients:

- ✓ 3 tbsp unsweetened cocoa powder
- ✓ ¼ cup erythritol

- ❖ Fill muffin pans and freeze for 3 hours until firm.

AUTHOR BIBLIOGRAPHY

THE PALEO DIET FOR MEN: The Guide with 150+ Grain- and Gluten-Free Recipes to Lose Weight and Start Whole-Foods Lifestyle!

THE PALEO DIET FOR WOMEN: 120+ Recipes to Discover the Secrets of Rapid Weight Loss and A Healthy Lifestyle Using the Paleo Diet!

THE PALEO DIET COOKBOOK: 120+ Tasty and Wholesome Recipes that Combine Paleo and Vegan Diet to Eating Well, Lose Weight, and Feeling Vibrant!

THE PALEO DIET FOR KIDS: 120+ Ultimate Paleo Recipes All Kid-Friendly to Become a Superheroes! All Paleo and Healthy -Based Food!

THE PALEO DIET FOR BEGINNERS: The Unique Guide to The Paleo Diet: 120+ Easy Recipes to Make Paleo Cooking Easy! regain your energy today!

THE PALEO DIET FOR COUPLE: THE SECRETS OF RAPID WEIGHT LOSS AND A HEALTHY LIFESTYLE USING THE PALEO DIET!

200+ Wholesome, Easy to Follow and Delicious Recipes!

CONCLUSIONS

The Paleo diet is a lifestyle answer that is steadily gaining popularity these days. Many people are finding this diet very beneficial to their health. It is a natural diet that focuses on whole and unprocessed foods.

With the Paleo diet, you can lose weight and feel healthier. The Paleo diet is low in sugar. It is free of grains, dairy, legumes, refined carbohydrates, and processed foods. This means you will eat natural foods rich in vitamins, minerals, antioxidants, and fiber.

The Paleo diet helps in the prevention of various diseases. Some benefits of the Paleo diet include an improved immune system and a reduced chance of developing cancer and heart disease. The Paleo diet is a way of eating that became popular in the early 2000s. It is a lifestyle that hunter-gatherers practiced for millions of years before agriculture. One of the key ideas is that we have evolved to eat foods that are in season. It's a way to ensure we get nutrients from our food. A simple way to implement this way of eating is to find whole, fresh foods in season. The Paleo diet does not encourage processed foods, fast foods, or refined sugars or oils. It is considered ideal for keeping the mind and body healthy. It encourages the consumption of fresh foods and minimizes exposure to chemicals such as preservatives and artificial additives. The Paleo diet is a way of life for Paleolithic humans. This means that the way they ate differed from the way we eat today. This diet is designed to mimic the eating habits of our ancestors. The Paleo diet focuses on eating foods that are rich in vitamins and minerals. These foods include fish, meat, vegetables, fruits, nuts, and seeds. This diet also encourages low glycaemic index fruits and vegetables.

As beneficial as this diet can be to your health, it also has drawbacks. For example, individuals who follow the Paleo diet may suffer from nutrient deficiencies. This type of diet can also lead to a higher incidence of health problems such as acne and cancer.

However, you address these issues, you need to know what the Paleo diet is and how it is used today.

Lightning Source UK Ltd.
Milton Keynes UK
UKHW050709110521
383453UK00002B/137